A PLACE TO LIVE

A Place to Live

Families and Child Health in a Cairo Neighborhood

Belgin Tekçe

Linda Oldham

Frederic Shorter

The American University in Cairo Press

113 Sharia Kasr el Aini
Cairo, Egypt

Dar el Kutub No. 3194/93
ISBN 977 424 315 3

Printed in Egypt at the Printshop of the American University in Cairo

Contents

Illustrations

Tables

Figures

Acknowledgments

Many people helped us bring this book to realization. The genesis of the idea owes much to the encouragement and support of Youssef el-Rafai, Chairman of the Executive Agency for Joint Projects (EAJP) of the Ministry of Housing at the time we planned and undertook this study. The EAJP is the agency responsible for urban area upgrading in Egypt and the sponsor of the survey in the community of Manshiet Nasser which is a primary source for this book. Eng. el-Rafai personally gave generously of his time for discussion of objectives and issues, and for the formalization of permissions necessary for such research in Egypt. We hope that he and others in the urban management professions will find this work a constructive contribution to the continuing dialogue about policies for the new communities.

Among the many others, we also wish to thank the following: W. Henry Mosley, Mounir Neamatalla, John Gerhart, and the late Ehsan Shiri for encouragement and suggestions at the early planning stages; Hussein Tamaa, Haguer el-Hadidi, Asma El Hakim, Nerman El Hiny, Eman Mohamed Ahmed, Safah Ferghali, Nagwa Amin, Heba Gaafer, Maha Sabet, and Magdi Tamaa for enthusiastic contributions to field work; Bruce MacLeod, Denise Batani, and Hani Hanna for data management; Hoda Rashad and Sahar el-Tawila for exceptional assistance with statistical questions; and for critical reading of part or all of the manuscript, Osman Galal, John Waterbury, Huda Zurayk, Ragui Assaad, Gail Harrison, Alan Duben, Janet Molzan, Dan Tschirgi, and participants in two Study Groups of the Middle East Research Awards Program in Population and Development (MEAwards).

In addition, we want to note the special hospitality and friendship that comes with the Egyptian way of life. The people of the Manshia gave generously by allowing us to observe their lives and to talk with them about themselves and their children. There were also many others in Cairo who learned of our work and helped us with it both professionally and personally.

The field study of Manshiet Nasser was carried out by staff of Environmental Quality International (EQI) of Cairo under the guidance of its president, Mounir Neamatalla, and EQI's director of research, Linda Oldham. Technical support was given by the regional office of The Population Council in Cairo and the Middle East Awards Program in Population and Development (MEAwards) headed by Frederic Shorter.

Financial support was provided by EQI and the Council, as well as by the Ford Foundation and the International Development Research Centre of Canada through the Middle East Research Awards Program in Population and Development (MEAwards).

ONE

The Setting and the Approach

Cairo's Unstoppable Growth

Cairo was already an important center of power and influence in its time and place a millennium ago. In the twentieth century it is one of the key regional centers of the world, foremost among Arab centers and the leading metropolis of the Middle East and North Africa. Today, its scale is almost double that of Istanbul or Tehran; one must travel as far west as London or east as Bombay to find another city of similar or greater size and complexity. The people who live in Cairo are at the heart of Egypt, drawn from the provincial cultures of Upper, Middle, and Lower Egypt, and amalgamated with generations of Cairenes to produce a mosaic of class and culture that is Cairo's very own.

In almost every era, starting from its earliest beginnings, Cairo has been a crowded city so far as its native quarters are concerned. Only the grand projects of an age of foreign domination and foreign residents, epitomized by the Khedive Ismail's projects in the latter half of the nineteenth century, were exceptions. Historically, the city did not claim a vast area and then fill it in slowly over hundreds of years. The area was small to begin with, and when more space was needed, it was found by pushing out the boundaries. The banks of the Nile were taken, after being made safe by stabilization of the river's channel and by drainage projects. The river level was brought under control by upstream barrages and reservoirs. Land development companies also expanded the city by claiming the desert on the perimeters of Cairo.[1]

During the present century, a great deal of rich agricultural land has disappeared beneath buildings as the city has grown, nearly always violating laws that were intended to protect the precious agricultural resource. The development policies of President Gamal 'Abd al-Nasser in the 1950s and 1960s brought large industrial projects to the north and south of the city, originally seen as satellites, but today they are part of the contiguous areal span of metropolitan Cairo. As Egypt has grown, so has Cairo, at times even faster as the city was boosted by migration from the provinces. From a country of ten million in 1900, Egypt became one of fifty-two million by 1990 and Cairo itself passed the marker of ten million.

Growth by migration

There was a tremendous spurt in Cairo's growth during and after the Second World War, triggered by interruptions in international trade and in particular by the Allied blockade of Europe which suddenly raised the demand for local provisions to serve urban populations and Allied troops stationed in Egypt and the Levant. Economic historian Charles Issawi notes, for example, that Allied troop expenditures equaled 25–30 percent of national income in Egypt, Palestine, and Lebanon during the Second World War (1982:161). Migrants from the provinces streamed into Cairo and other Delta cities, responding to opportunities in small-scale workshops, commerce, and services. In addition, Egypt was on the eve of a transformation of its own economy that would see decades of expansion in several branches of the economy such as government, manufacturing, trade, and eventually tourism,

Table 1-1. The population of Egypt and Cairo, 1897–2000

	Population in Thousands		Cairo as a percentage of Egypt
Censuses	Egypt	Cairo[a]	
1897	9,635	905	9.4
1907	11,190	1,071	9.6
1917	12,718	1,254	9.9
1927	14,178	1,572	11.1
1937	15,921	1,893	11.9
1947	18,967	2,779	14.7
1960	25,984	4,530	17.5
1976	36,626	7,471	20.4
1986	48,205	9,754	20.2
Projection			
2000	65,000	13,000	20.0

a. Cairo is defined as in the 1986 Egyptian census report, literally translated as 'Cairo urban sprawl'. The time series is constructed to hold the 1986 definition constant and thus to offer comparable figures. Nevertheless, higher estimates are often given for the present population and could be supported by the following reasoning: ten years earlier, in 1976, the census office used a larger areal definition of metropolitan Cairo. That definition adds about 670,000 people to the 1976 figure, and would add about 1,000,000 to the 1986 estimate. It is often pointed out that the daytime population is greater because it includes commuters from other towns and villages.

Sources: CAPMAS (1978; 1987), Preliminary Master Plan of 1970 cited in Aga Khan Award (1985), and Shorter (1989:4-5).

that would shift the national deployment of the labor force in favor of the cities, i.e. urbanization. Cairo was a main recipient of the shift.

During the decades following the Second World War, migration continued with new sources of propulsion to replace those that faded with the end of the war. Poor conditions in agriculture and increasing population pressure on the land made the comparison of living in the provinces with life in Cairo appear advantageous to the latter, so people moved. Furthermore, the new socialist society of Nasser offered educational opportunities and public sector employment in Cairo. One more factor that entered the equation was the general decline in death rates in Egypt that raised the pressure of population growth throughout the country.

These were the years when an increasing proportion of Egyptians made their homes in Cairo; the percentage living in Cairo rose from a pre-war 12 percent to 20 percent by the 1970s (Table 1-1). The relative importance of Cairo as the place to live and work rose steadily until the 1973 war. Major changes in the regional economy suddenly imposed themselves and these affected the flow of Egyptians into Cairo. The oil exporting countries of the Gulf (and Libya) became super-rich as oil prices remained high after the war, granting to those countries vastly increased revenues. As rich countries they needed the poor and the not-so-poor to build and staff their development projects and to meet their demand for every kind of social and personal services. For Egyptians, this set in motion massive emigration abroad for work. Egyptian families in the provinces could send family members, chiefly males, abroad to realize projects of preparation for marriage, income to live better, or to raise capital for housing or business. They did not need to move from provincial towns and villages to Cairo either as a preparatory step upon return to pursue their ambitions.

The ladder of economic advance that depends upon migrating for work abroad is still in place, though it was shown to have high risks by the Gulf War in 1991. More than a million Egyptians returned home, most of them suffering serious uncompensated financial and professional losses. International politics is a factor that frequently upsets the employment system in this part of the world. Since then, there has been a revival of work opportunities in the Gulf, but the prospects for work both at home and abroad have run out of steam. Since the mid-1980s real wages have lost their buoyancy, and declined in some sectors, against a background of increasing pressure from faster growth in the labor force than in job opportunities.

The relevance of this for Cairo's growth by migration is that no sudden increase in propulsion of population from the provinces has happened or indeed may be expected to overwhelm Cairo in the immediate future as it once did. Furthermore, there are now other major cities in the Delta that receive a share of the urban growth by migration.

Cairo's history as a place to move to when provincial Egyptians are young and mobile has left its mark. Old-family Cairenes often remark on how the city has become a 'city of peasants,' *fellahin* from the Delta and *saidi*s from Upper Egypt. Cairo is truly a city that reflects the provinces, incorporating many of the ways that people live in smaller towns and in villages. Practically everyone living in the provinces has a relative or an acquaintance in Cairo, and the network is mobilized when needed. Aspects of provincial culture—a term we prefer because it connotes more than agricultural ways of life—are interwoven with each other and with urban ways to develop distinctively Cairene styles of life. The numerous subcultures that this produces in Cairo have both class and regional characteristics to which we must be sensitive.

Numerically, however, migration is no longer a major source of growth. Most Cairenes are at least second-generation, more often third or more. A comparative statistic helps to make the point. Cairo is inhabited only to the extent of 19 percent by persons who were born somewhere else, whereas another major regional city that is truly growing by migration, Istanbul, is inhabited to the extent of 60 percent by people who moved there from somewhere else.[2] Thus, to understand Cairo's growth in recent decades, and the momentum that will almost certainly maintain its growth in the immediate future, one must examine the internal dynamics of family reproduction in the city.

Growth by family reproduction

The usual approach to a discussion of natural increase is to follow the trends of births minus deaths, which provide a numerical 'explanation' for that source of city growth. We shall take a different line, and look at family multiplication in Cairo as it has changed over time. That will bring to the fore the family-level process of social and biological reproduction that produces the demographic aggregates of births and deaths.

Cairo's families have been participating in a collective transition from relatively high mortality and fertility toward lower and lower levels for some time. This is seen in Table 1-2. The crude birth and death rates are complemented by refined indices for fertility and mortality. These indices are not affected by the peculiarities of age structure that influence levels and trends in the crude rates. Total fertility per woman in the table is the number of births that women are currently having; it is the sum of births across the entire reproductive period based on current age-specific birth rates. The downward trends in mortality and fertility are persistent and have not been reversed, so one can be quite sure that a genuine and strong demographic transition is in progress.[3]

The demographic transition is a general one in Egypt, less advanced in Upper Egypt and more so in Lower Egypt. The urban–rural differentials, in

Table 1-2. Trends of fertility and mortality in Cairo, 1960–2000

Five-year periods	Crude rates per 1000			Refined indices		
	Births	Deaths	Natural increase	Total fertility per woman	Infant mortality per 1000 births	Expectation of life at birth (years)
Actual						
1960-1965	43.1	15.9	27.2	5.72	160.9	50.6
1965-1970	37.1	14.2	22.8	4.81	152.3	51.9
1970-1975	34.6	12.8	21.7	4.33	137.6	53.6
1975-1980	35.6	10.4	25.2	4.15	102.8	58.9
1980-1985	32.5	8.8	23.7	3.79	75.6	62.0
1985-1990	28.0	6.8	21.3	3.37	45.6	65.0
Projections						
1990-1995	23.4	6.2	17.2	3.00	32.6	67.3
1995-2000	20.8	6.0	14.7	2.66	28.0	69.6
Year 2000	20.2	5.9	14.3	2.52	25.8	70.5

Technical note: The estimates of actual values and the projections are prepared on the basis of vital registration and census data for the Cairo urban region. Population simulations are used to transform the data into consistent time series for each variable and to make the projections. Comparisons with estimates from additional sources (surveys and special studies) were also used to confirm the general validity of the estimates. For details, see Shorter (1989:10-12).

favor of urban, are not large region by region. What is happening in Cairo demographically is remarkably like the general average for Egypt as a whole. No doubt this is due in some measure to the presence in Cairo of families at many different stages of the transition, some advanced, others not.

Infant mortality has fallen phenomenally. Together with gains in adult survival there is now a much higher expectation of life at birth than formerly. The medical services and the educational media, especially television, claim that much of the credit for the accelerated decline in infant and child mortality of the 1980s (Table 1-2) should go to heightened awareness of effective technologies for home (or clinic) treatment of diarrheal disease and their adoption.[4] Whatever the reasons, families have revised radically what they expect relative to the survival of their families. Most children will now survive to adulthood and this is known. Women waste far less time on unsuccessful pregnancies, deliveries, and disappointing struggles to keep young children healthy and alive.

Another improvement in prospects is a reduced fear of mobilization and war. Peace is never a certain thing, but Egyptians in the 1980s had much more of a sense than they did in the 1960s that the family will not lose members by long absence or fatalities and disabilities over which they would have no control. The public safety net of subsidized basic foods and health care services, despite many shortcomings, is another factor that provides a sense of security.

For all these reasons, bringing up children has become a responsibility with continuity, less likely to be shaken by tragic losses. That makes many births less necessary and each birth more expensive. The cost of children in terms of care, time, and money has risen. Looming as an increasingly important problem is the expense of education for children, which until recently was theoretically provided free, but has long been expensive in practice. Fees for schools, for uniforms, and for books and supplies, plus the cost of tutoring are now serious costs. At a time when families are striving to put all their children through the lower levels of school and some of them all the way to university level, this is one more cost deterrent to bearing additional children. As we trace out the changes in the family over the last thirty or forty years, others that contribute to the smaller family norm come forward.[5]

Women's roles have become more complex and multi-faceted. Part of this is participation along with their husbands in a new consumerism that has seized all classes, even including the lower classes of Cairo since the 1970s. Consumer trends have been fueled by money from the Gulf states and encouraged by extensive media and marketing relations with foreign companies under the open-door (*infitah*) policy.

Other important factors include educational opportunities for women that first became important in the Nasser period. This led to more commitment of girls as well as boys to school. Schooling has become a valued goal of families in Cairo. It is a gateway to advancement of social position and economic returns through employment. For boys, this does not always pay off, and many leave school early to be apprenticed and make more money in workshops and trade. For girls, to have an education has become an important asset, virtually with a cash value, when seeking a marriage partner (MacLeod, 1991; Singerman, 1989).

Recent research, though based on studies in Mexico, suggests links that could well be operative in the Cairene setting as well. LeVine (1991) has shown that women's schooling experience contributes to reduced fertility and child mortality through a number of intervening psychosocial characteristics acquired through schooling, apart from its effects on status enhancement and improved access to employment opportunities. These include ideational changes in aspirations about self and children, in parental investment strategies, and the development of a new kind of mother-child relationship with the result that child rearing becomes a more labor consuming activity for educated mothers.

In the early stages of fertility control in Egypt, couples relied on folk methods, including withdrawal, and pregnancy termination by abortion.[6] The desire for control increased at about the same time as modern medical means of contraception became available in Egypt, so these methods have largely displaced the folk methods and account for most of the increase in fertility regulation. Since the mid-1950s, Egypt has had an on-again off-again national policy in favor of contraception supported by media campaigns and public provisioning of contraceptive devices and services. In recent years, the state policy has been consistently favorable and much international assistance has been lavished on the program. To what extent this has been a motivating factor or simply a facilitating one is impossible to assess. However, it is presently possible in Cairo to find a range of contraceptive services and materials at reasonable costs, even though the options and services continue to attract criticism.

The net result of these changes in childbearing is an average of about three births per family in Cairo at present, down from about six when the Republic was established in 1952. The improvement of child and young adult survival needs to be taken into account as well, in order to follow the trend of surviving children, since it is the survivors who grow up and eventually form new households. In this connection, it is helpful to turn to an index demographers use, the net reproduction rate.

Formally, the net reproduction rate shows how many daughters will survive to the mid-point of childbearing, given the fertility and mortality rates prevailing at the time of their birth. In plain language, with reasonable assumptions about when women marry and the assumption that virtually all of them do marry, the net reproduction rate gives the rate of multiplication of couples who will eventually form new families passing from generation to generation over time. Mortality assumptions are part of the calculation of the net reproduction rate, allowing for the demise of individuals by infant, child, and young adult mortality before they can contribute personally to the perpetual process of population renewal.

In Table 1-3, we see that the net reproduction rate was 2.0 in the early 1960s. It fell about one-fourth up to 1990 and is clearly on a downward trajectory.[7] When, and if, it reaches 1.0, there would only be replacement and no multiplication of the number of families. For each new couple that starts a family there is not necessarily a new and separate household, but as we are going to show below, the numerical equivalence between the net reproduction rate and the multiplication of households in Cairo is close.

While this bit of demographic logic would seem to say that the main surge toward the formation of new households came in the 1960s and therefore is past history, that is far from true. There is a time lapse between birth and

Table 1-3. Household multiplication: How the current net reproduction rate affects the formation of new families in the next generation

Period of birth of a female birth cohort	Prevailing net reproduction rate (multiplier for new families)	Time (one generation later) when the female birth cohort will form new families[a]
1960-1965	2.04	1985
1965-1970	1.75	1990
1970-1975	1.62	1995
1975-1980	1.68	2000
1980-1985	1.61	2005
1985-1990	1.52	2010
Projection		
1990-1995	1.38	2015
1995-2000	1.24	2020
2000-2005	1.12	2025

a. The dating of these multipliers is based on the assumption that the mean age of marriage of females is between 20 and 25 years and that all females who survive to adulthood marry.

marriage. The impact of the net reproduction rate prevailing 'today' is felt as a demand for housing only twenty or twenty-five years later, corresponding with the time it takes for girls to grow to adulthood, marry, and start their own families. Some of the couples that are formed never contribute to the multiplication of households, because they live with the parental generation or succeed them in the old dwellings. However, in Cairo, unlike the countryside, only a small fraction of the newly formed families fail to establish independent homes.[8]

For each cohort of women that is born, we can date the time when they will form families of their own, which are the dates written in the last column of Table 1-3. Only females need to be tracked in this exercise, because each female will form a new family in her adulthood (with husband of course). When the multiplier says there will be two new families, it means that the number of families will double, and together with their children they will require housing.

These calculations are valuable to show that the force of new demand for living space that comes from the resident Cairo population was not only strong in the mid-1980s (first line of Table 1-3), but will remain strong well into the twenty-first century. Although the size of the multiplier is declining, simple replacement of one generation's families by the next is a long way off.

Additional new households are created when migrant families, usually young adults, arrive in Cairo to set up homes for themselves. Thus, there are two deviations from the pure multiplication of the net reproduction rate, which have opposite (offsetting) effects. One is the permanent doubling up of new families in parent households, which reduces the multiplier. The other is additions by migration, which increases it. As we have argued, neither of these is currently a major factor. Consequently, rates of multiplication in households are currently close to the appropriately-dated net reproduction rate.

In the twenty-six years between the 1960 and 1986 censuses, the number of households in Cairo more than doubled, adding more than one million new households to be located somewhere. This observed doubling confirms the explanation we have offered. The multiplier in Table 1-3 was also approximately two or slightly higher over that same interval of time.[9] Consequently, it is no wonder that there seems to be a limitless supply of young Cairene families looking for a place to live.

New settlements

The force of family reproduction is being absorbed by three-dimensional growth in Cairo's physical dimensions. Space is being created by expanding existing structures, by spilling over into surrounding areas, and by shrinking the size of home accommodations. Upward expansion occurs when additional floors are added to buildings, or the roof itself is used for makeshift dwellings on top. For many families, the first choice if they own a building is to add a floor, and allocate dwelling units to their children when they start their own families. Some buildings simply grow outward, becoming fatter, adding more units, which themselves may be no more than a single room, covering the ground space between buildings. Some of the additions are strictly commercial, not family projects, offering space for sale or rent with a substantial payment up front.

Second, the city spreads outward onto agricultural land, desert, or hillsides. These are the new settlements. They vary from orderly development projects to incursions without benefit of legality. The map (Figure 1-1) shows by two heavy dotted lines the historical limit of watered (agricultural) land on either side of the Nile. The city has expanded since 1947 onto vast areas of this agricultural land—it was already using some of it—as well as onto the desert to the northeast and east. The official urban development strategy for Cairo favors expansion into the desert, led by prior placement of infrastructure. But agricultural land already has some kind of water if not good sewerage, and people cannot wait.

Occasionally, enclaves that have somehow survived within the city are developed for housing, or in rare instances a seriously decayed area is redeveloped. Such ventures also expand the habitable space, even if they do not push out the perimeter of the city. On the map, one sees numerous unbuilt spaces, more of them toward the edges, many of which will be occupied in the future.

The expansion process as it actually unfolds absorbs land in three ways, not all of them condoned by the urban planners. One type is more or less planned and controlled development, another is uncontrolled building on private land (almost always agricultural land), and the third is uncontrolled squatting on state land. The last nearly always involves tacit permission of the authorities, but remains illegal.

The third dimension is to cram more people into existing space by subdivision of old dwelling units and to build smaller units as more and more new buildings go up. Such is the demand of young families for separate housing, that they sacrifice on standards of space and are steady customers for such units. Of course, there is also luxury housing, but it seldom achieves the spacious, high-ceiling design of flats of old. Those historic flats that remain are the prized possessions of families who for one reason or another, usually because of rent control, have been able to hold on, and who try to pass them down to their children. The threat to them is demolition and replacement by high-rise buildings, at a large profit to building contractors.

The built environment which has been created as a result of this three-dimensional growth in urban space has been produced largely through informal processes. Informality is a term frequently used in the urban literature, particularly in relation to the urban economy, but also for urban housing. A great diversity of meanings is attached to the term. At the most general level informality is used to refer to a process which is 'unregulated by the institutions of society in a legal and social environment in which similar activities are regulated.'[10] Thus, the boundaries of informality are highly context specific and historically fluid. Whether and what aspects of land acquisition and housing construction may be considered informal depends upon the regulations governing such activities at any point in time in a specific urban setting.

Different degrees of informality exist, because each particular case may involve single or multiple contraventions of law concerning ownership, land use, or building regulations. In Cairo, builders may purchase agricultural land legally, or already have title, but land use regulations prohibit residential building. Desert land raises the problem that it is not made available for legal construction until infrastructure has been placed, and that condition is seldom fulfilled in time. At each step there are boundaries between formally legal and informal building, which make it likely that much of the new building will be informal for one reason or another.

Eighty percent of the dwelling units built in Cairo since 1970 are in one respect or another informal according to a well-regarded study carried out in 1980 (Abt Associates, 1982). Among other things, this statistic raises the issue of whether a distinction between formal and informal housing is useful when regulations governing the construction of housing seem not to be well institutionalized. The same study points out, however, that the proportion informal has oscillated over time with informal provisioning expanding and shrinking in different historical periods. When all dwelling units in the study are considered, going back as far as the 1950s and 1960s, the proportion informal averages 62 percent (p.32). This suggests that the distinction is well worth maintaining in analysis of the organization of urban life in Cairo.

Informality should not be immediately identified with an absence of structural standards or with poverty. The informal communities of Cairo, far from being shantytowns such as those depicted in the urban literature on many Third World cities, are largely composed of sturdy brick structures, often reaching three to six stories high. People have built outside the law because there was rarely any other option, and their needs had to be met somehow. This solution has, of course, brought many problems, since communities could become established without minimal infrastructure or services and have crowded layouts or dense intermingling of incompatible land uses. A great deal of construction by and for the middle and upper classes has proceeded equally outside the building laws, but usually with more success at locating on land serviced by infrastructure. Thus, informality should not be identified solely with migrants and lower-class inhabitants, but with builders in every class. This even includes the old parts of Cairo where additions, demolitions, and rebuilding have often proceeded informally, bringing problems of substandard construction, loss of open space, and overloading of infrastructure.

Nevertheless, many communities have been established and vast masses of people have been housed through these legally invisible processes. From a Cairene lower-middle or lower class perspective, the new settlements are 'nice places to live.' The present study sets out to investigate how 'nice' by studying the implications for human welfare of the organization of community and household life in one of these settlements.

The community we have chosen to study, Manshiet Nasser, reflects in many ways the dynamics of the new settlements in Cairo, but each also has its own distinctive history (see map, location code 1). There is usually a special story to explain the initial settlement of the neighborhood, involving people displaced from some other location, or the first moves are due to the entrepreneurial initiative of a few families on the spot who function as developers. The mode of initial settlement affects the subsequent development of the community's character. In many instances, where the settlement occupies vacant desert or hillside land, as in Manshiet Nasser, there is a core of local political and social cohesion from the start. It is imported by the first settlers who adapt the structures of social support they knew in their places of origin. When the settlement is on private agricultural lands the organization of political and social life usually grows out of the community's earlier structure as a village. However, the new residents, especially if they come in large numbers from other subcultures of the city, may not be drawn in and fail to find supportive networks.[11] Some settlements succeed in creating communities, others do not.

Whatever the starting point, changes occur in community governance and in the social networks, as the settlements become large, and their politico-social systems are overpowered by the many problems that follow from density and variation in the origins of newcomers. In studying specific communities, one needs to locate the picture one obtains at the time of the study within the developmental sequence of the settlement itself. Over time, integration into the Cairo urban system proceeds and solutions are found to old problems while new ones emerge as part of the process of becoming recognized and subordinated to the larger system.

The particular community that we shall be studying in depth includes a considerable variety of people in terms of regional and class origins, and varieties of class aspirations. Yet the community is identified in the fabric of Cairo as being Upper Egyptian in regional origin and culture. When income levels and occupational characteristics are used as markers of class position, the community belongs to the lower part of the urban class structure. It is lower-middle and lower class in the social hierarchy, but with a strong presence of upwardly mobile craft and small scale business people. The people of this settlement are tied much more to private business and informal economic structures, and less to the public-sector government employment systems that were so popular and had their origin in the pre-Sadat, Nasser socialist period.

Health as a Component and Indicator of Human Welfare

For the study of Manshiet Nasser we wanted a concept that would capture important aspects of human welfare. No pretension of dealing comprehensively with the meaning and measurement of human welfare is intended. Ours was a deep interest in the quality of life of people in the new neighborhoods, and curiosity about the ability of the social sciences to enrich understanding of the determinants of the particular level of welfare that the people achieve. Several lines of thinking led us to choose infant and child health as a measure of human welfare in the new settlements of Cairo. This would become the outcome measure that would guide the design of our field research and our investigation of the determinants of welfare, represented by children's health.

At the time this research was undertaken in the mid-1980s, measures of income or of production (which generates income) were under attack as inadequate indices of development and of achieved standards of living. By extension, the criticisms first made at the national level of assessment also apply to measurements at community and household levels. While no one really doubted the value of measuring national income or national product, these measures had shortcomings. Women's work both inside and outside the home was not captured. There was more to development and the achievement of a standard of living than the volume of material goods or services. There were also questions of just and unjust distribution, environmental impact, and whether people were really living in a better way or not.

In the scurry to fix things up, one of the indices that became popular was the expectation of life, or simply the infant mortality rate. Attempts were made to combine these and other indices—such as educational levels—with the economic measures. New ways were devised to credit women with more production, though many of them foundered at the implementation stage. The main line of attack was to observe and measure more of the non-economic aspects of the social system, and thus to create a more comprehensive social accounting system. The basket was enlarged, items were weighted and summed together, and new overall indices were put forward. The most recent in this genre is the 'human development index' which combines three types of information: gross national product, literacy and years of schooling, and the average expectation of life at birth (UN Development Programme, 1991).[12]

In principle, there is no difficulty in taking these national concepts down to a household level, so long as we may group households in meaningful clusters for analysis. The key issue is whether the concepts measure human welfare, or at least some important aspect of it.

Economic activity by household members brings income, but is not itself a measure of the household's welfare. Income is used for daily household activities that support life: feeding, sheltering, clothing, recreating, educating, and so on. No doubt more income makes for more welfare, but not unambiguously and not without conditions. Income is one of the means of acquiring inputs that the household transforms into the outputs of human welfare. Something similar can be said of the educational endowments that members of the household have. Direct enjoyment of being educated, without further transformation, no doubt exists, but an important function of this personal resource is instrumental. The educational experience contributes to the household members' ability to produce welfare in the household, but not unconditionally.

The expectation of life at birth is a completely different kind of index. It summarizes the mortality experience of a group of people across the entire life course; thus, it is a measure of the standard of health that a group, or population, experiences. If health is a major element of human welfare, which we consider it to be, then the expectation of life is a measure of welfare output. Better health may also contribute to economic productivity, but its first meaning is that it describes important welfare consequences of the day to day living processes in a particular setting.

As we study households and their functioning we shall separate inputs from outputs of the household's activities. The income that household members earn, including the production of valuable goods and services by women, will be conceptualized as inputs. So will the educational endowments of members of the household. And there will be other inputs in the conceptual framework for this study. In addition, the structure and functioning of the household as the institution within which much of the production of the health output is achieved, will be examined.

There was a time in the development of economic theory when the household was regarded as an end point, or consumer, of national production; it's complex processes of transformation of inputs into outputs could be left mysteriously behind the walls of family privacy. It was not an institution within the socioeconomic system whose performance was assessed by the indices. While this is still true to an alarming extent, new interests have come to the foreground. It has taken the nagging of other disciplines and innovators from within economics itself to redefine boundaries and explore the new interests.

These new interests concern how the family participates in production, how it functions with regard to pooling and distribution of valuable things, how it is managed, the roles of different members as they are delineated by gender and stage of the life course, and the way in which their options in the society at large affect the internal workings of families. Internal dynamics of families are an integral part of the processes that produce good or ill health in children.

For our measure of welfare, we will be using the health of infants and young children. Mortality rates, and summaries such as the expectation of life at birth, are all useful measures of health. One of the characteristics of mortality rates at different ages is that they are strongly associated statistically with each other. Lower rates at early ages co-exist with lower rates at all ages above childhood.[13] This allows us to say that measures of child health are indicators by proxy of health at all ages, hence of the entire study population.

This is not just a statistical piece of luck. The predominant causes of death vary from childhood diseases to old-age diseases, but the social and environmental conditions of life, which are shared by the young and old, seem to affect all ages, albeit through different disease etiologies. A community with good medical services for adults will usually have them also for children; good food supply usually benefits both; technological choices that minimize accidents are likely to be present, or absent as the case may be, at all ages. The family that looks after its older members well is likely to do the same for mothers during pregnancy and childbirth, and to help its children develop in a healthy manner. None of these uniformities is absolute, but the tendencies are strong.

Finally, and this is perhaps the most important reason why death rates at different ages are correlated with each other, is that death is increasingly understood by the health sciences to be the cumulative consequence of patterns of everyday living, rather than due to specific, critical, disease episodes. The final events, or causes of death are only the end points for the longer, cumulative processes. This applies across all ages and for a range of levels of general mortality. We do not want to make too strong a case for the correlations by age, since that would suppress many details that lead to interesting conclusions in particular populations. However, the historical demographic evidence in national life tables is strongly consistent with this way of looking at health across different ages in any particular population.[14]

While we have thus far written of measures of health status solely in terms of mortality, additional approaches are also available and are used in this study. Among the living, a good general measure of health is nutritional status. This is assessed in the very young by anthropometric measurements, such as weight against a standard curve for growth in body mass, differentiating by sex. The word 'nutrition' is troublesome, because it is often used to describe diet, but it is also a physiological condition that results from a cluster of biological factors, including disease as well as diet.[15] It is in the sense of general physiological status, not diet, that we use the term 'nutritional status'. The prevalence of specific diseases, including parasites, are also subjects of the study.

Not included solely because the state of the art did not permit us to do so competently in a field survey, are assessments of child development at very young ages. Psychosocial and motor development in children contribute to physiological growth and are valuable welfare outcomes in themselves.[16] There is more to the meaning of health than physical survival and growth alone, and child development certainly deserves attention both as an objective and as a means to better child survival, even if it was not possible to make the relevant measurements and observations in the present study.[17]

Layered Inquiry: From Urban Structures to Health

The logic of inquiry for this study proceeds from an examination of urban structures of daily life through the connecting links that finally produce levels of human welfare represented by child health. The framework is basically rather simple, although complexities arise as it is implemented in analysis. The book itself is organized by chapters to reveal and investigate the layers that ultimately lead to health outcomes. The central theme is that social context, represented by the organization of life in the community, in households, and among members of the household, consistently bear upon the quality of health that is achieved.

We take the position that there is far more to health than medicine and medical practice, and our intention is to bring this out carefully and with as much testing of its validity as possible. While doing so, the important linkage between the urban social system, practices at the family level, and physiological outcomes for children must be filled in rigorously, because health is the result of a bio-social process. To illustrate the point by a simple statement, children do not live or die because their families are rich or poor; there is a whole system of processes that translate being rich or poor into food, exposure risks, disease, treatment, and so on, which have biological effects on children. Yet children do live or die because their families are rich or poor! For the variable 'rich or poor', many others could be substituted to illustrate the reasoning.

As social scientists, we have borrowed heavily, and learned much, from the health sciences. A particularly helpful research framework has been the Mosley–Chen one on the relationship of a set of 'intermediate' variables to health (1984). These are such variables as dietary patterns, age of the child, susceptibility to disease, exposure, treatment practices, and others. Their outcome variable is child survival (mortality rates). Among the determinants of these intermediate variables is a black box of social factors whose existence is recognized by their framework, but it stops short of investigating the contents and explaining the role of these factors. One can view the present study as a contribution to filling that box with more meaning. To the extent that we have succeeded, the results should be of interest to health scientists who wish to learn more about the social system within which their particular field of interest is situated.

The layered system is investigated first of all by taking a brief look at the processes by which new settlements are created in Cairo. Driving the process is a system of family reproduction, a system which itself is changing rapidly in Cairo as family lifestyles change. To convey the idea of what family reproduction means in the Cairene context, we may pause to recount the story of one young couple's solution as they embark on their own family cycle. This illustration comes from Arlene MacLeod's field work in Cairo (personal communication, 1988).

Karima is a married woman in her early thirties. She and her husband both work in clerical positions in government offices in a large building in the center of Cairo. Their occupation raises their prestige sufficiently to make them part of the lower-middle class, but their income makes this status quite tenuous. Karima grew up in Sayyida Zeinab (an old area of Cairo), and her widowed mother still lives in her rent-controlled flat of two tiny rooms. Karima and her husband searched the area for a home before they married, but discovered the impossibility of finding an affordable place to live near her family. They were very disappointed as they regard the areas outside Sayyida Zeinab as less friendly and less desirable. They finally located an affordable flat in a neighborhood of Dar al-Salam (see map, location code 8), which is a large new settlement built on private agricultural land, and rented it. Each day they commute into the city to work.

The traffic and crowds are so troublesome that they leave their home very early each morning (about 4 A.M.) and travel to the house of Karima's mother with their two small children. The family then goes back to sleep for a couple of hours. About seven, they all get up and the parents depart for their offices, while the children remain for the day with Karima's mother. In the afternoon, Karima returns to fetch the children before continuing on to their home. There, she cleans and straightens up the house before beginning to cook the hot dinner. Her husband, who holds a second job in the afternoon, returns home about nine in the evening. This extra trip each day helps solve both the problems of childcare and the crowded commute to work.[18]

Just as Karima's family epitomizes the process of intra-city resettlement for one class group, hers being lower-middle class and Cairene, so it happens with other class and origin groups as well. Our own in-depth look at patterns of living in contemporary Cairo is through the window of Manshiet Nasser, also a relatively new neighborhood. This settlement is the main actor in our story and frames many of the questions and ideas that are pursued.

The urban literature is full of labels such as 'marginal,' 'squatter,' 'shanty,' 'informal,' and 'spontaneous' to refer to quarters of cities built largely by informal processes and presumed to be the habitations of the urban poor. Differences in terminology reflect different emphases and intellectual perspectives on Third World urbanization, and no one term is enough to describe all aspects of the dynamics of these settlements. We use the term 'self-help' from time to time to emphasize that such settlements are responses to many of the problems generated in peripheral economies under the pressure of population growth and limited resources, where economic and social needs outrun the capacity of formal public institutions to cope promptly and effectively with demands.

The institution which draws communal and individual resources together and supports daily life for its members is the family, and families are situated in households. In a broader sense families often extend over several households, sometimes close by and sometimes with considerable distance separating them from each other. For each family group that coresides there is a concentration and management of resources which affects the welfare of its members in a particularly immediate way. We see the household as the key social site for the production of welfare, in terms of child health. A chapter is devoted therefore to the formation and functioning of households in Manshiet Nasser. Cairo households as a whole are viewed from time to time in the chapter to distinguish what is characteristic of new settlements and what is general throughout the city.

Then a first look is taken at the relationship of household resources and functioning to child health. This is more of a question-raising than answering chapter. It asks why children die, but looks only at the social conditions, not the processes intermediate between those social conditions and the physiological welfare of children. In Manshiet Nasser the differential risks of death which children face are startling. They are not small differentials even though we are looking at only a single community that has a superficial appearance of being all the same. Clearly it is not. For Cairo as a whole, therefore, the differences in life chances for the newborn are even greater. By extension of the argument made earlier, this indicates that health differs greatly by social conditions for persons of all ages in the Cairo population.

To unfold the layers of relationships carefully, the ways in which recurrent infection and undernutrition weaken children in the specific context of Manshiet Nasser is investigated next. These are the intermediate processes that were mentioned earlier as part of the Mosley–Chen framework. The main argument is that weakening occurs in a cumulative and synergistic manner. The attention shifts in the course of the discussion from the etiology of particular diseases to social practices surrounding health or illness. We also see how elements of this process can be verified by statistical analysis using procedures familiar in the social sciences, but here applied to interaction of the biological and the social.

Among the most important factors affecting whether children are set on a 'road to health', to impaired life, or to death, is the quality of home management of health. The question is the maintenance of health and treatment of illness when required. A chapter is devoted to the home management of health, based partly on survey information, but also on in-depth observations as well. We consider the extent to which families have options, socially, not just technically, to improve conditions given the environment in which they live. To illustrate functioning at this layer of the analytic framework, contributions from researchers working in similar areas of Cairo are included.

All the layers are analytically connected, from the urban structures of life to the health outcome for children. At the end of the book different layers of the analysis are brought together, and the broad findings and some of their implications are discussed.

A Note on Data Sources

In the following chapters, we shall be drawing on many sources and using the results of several different procedures for direct observation in the field. We have been interested in the written history of Cairo, in novels that describe everyday life, and in scholarly studies. We have talked with many Cairenes who have themselves lived through the processes we are describing, or have observed them from their own perspectives. The authors have lived a

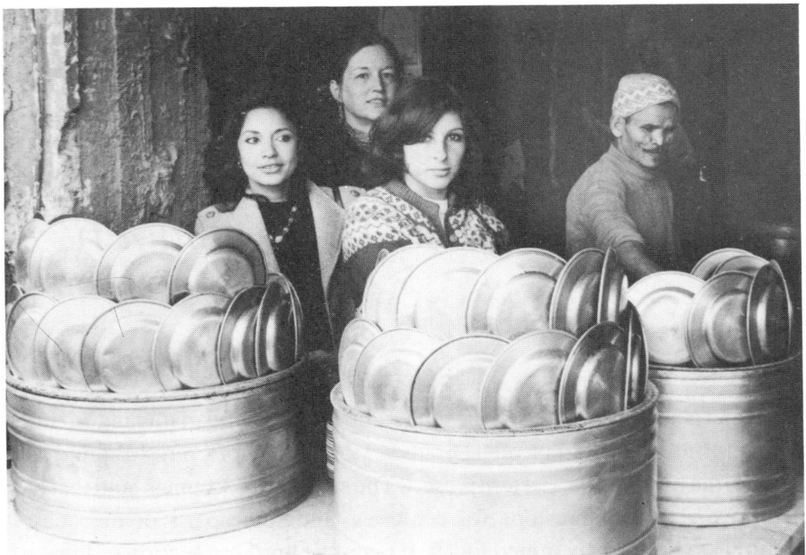

Team members in the field: koshari shop. Photograph by Nadir Hashem.

significant part of their own professional lives in Cairo: ten, twenty, and twelve years respectively.

The research for this book began in earnest with ethnographic field work, which was followed by a field survey conducted in the mid-1980s in Manshiet Nasser. We continued to visit the community from that time until this book went to press in the early 1990s, making additional observations, which, though less well documented, are nonetheless valid data. They help show the direction and pace of trends, for Manshiet Nasser, like all of Cairo, is a community in motion.

The main survey was a representative household survey. The frame for the survey was a complete census of plots and buildings carried out for the government's interdepartmental Joint Housing Projects Agency a few months beforehand. The sample was a systematic representative sample of dwelling units drawn from the lists of all buildings and dwelling units. Interviewing took place in March–April, 1984.

The survey instruments were a questionnaire for the household (N=1118), one for ever-married women under age fifty (N=962), and one for mothers about children aged less than three years (N=699). For children without mothers (N=2), the responsible person was interviewed. All the children under age three were weighed, and stool specimens were taken from a subsample aged 24–35 months (N=112). Fecal samples were examined for helminth ova and protozoan forms. Intensive ethnographic work was carried out prior to the construction of interview schedules, during the survey, and intermittently throughout the period of analysis and writing to the present time to provide interpretive information.

TWO

Manshiet Nasser: The Community

Setting

Manshiet Nasser is situated on the rocky slopes of the Muqattam range of hills which forms an eastern physical boundary to the city of Cairo.[1] Behind and beyond the hills lies the Eastern Desert. The settlement occupies land that has been quarried for limestone for centuries, and some parts of the quarry continue to be actively mined today. It faces the northern section of the vast Mamluk burial quarters, and beyond them it looks at the oldest and one of the most densely populated quarters of the city, the Gamaliya, including the historic bazaar and the al-Azhar quarters. Manshiet Nasser is separated from the medieval core of the city, only two kilometers away, by the cemetery areas. A newly built highway delineates where Manshiet Nasser ends and the cemeteries begin. There is also a single track rail line along this boundary of the settlement. Topography dictates the roughly rectangular shape of the settlement; the community is wedged between the cemetery on one side and the rugged cliffs rising above the settlement on the other. The total area of occupation is approximately 1.5 square kilometers.

A large community of garbage collectors, the Zabbaleen, occupies the top of the Muqattam hills, overlooking Manshiet Nasser. Members of this community collect household garbage in Cairo, transport it up the hill, sort, recycle, and sell its useful components. Many of the Zabbaleen travel down through Manshiet Nasser with their donkey carts early in the morning on their way to collect garbage, and return with loaded carts in the afternoon. They use land for animals, sorting yards, and storage, with a lower human settlement density than in Manshiet Nasser. The Zabbaleen are mostly Christians, while the neighboring residents of Manshiet Nasser below are predominantly Muslim. The pace of expansion is so rapid that the Zabbaleen community, which could be seen only at a distance in 1980, has now merged with Manshiet Nasser. At the boundaries, there is now a spillover of house renting, cross-overs for utilization of social services, and commercial intercourse—all on a limited scale but indicative of social blending as well.

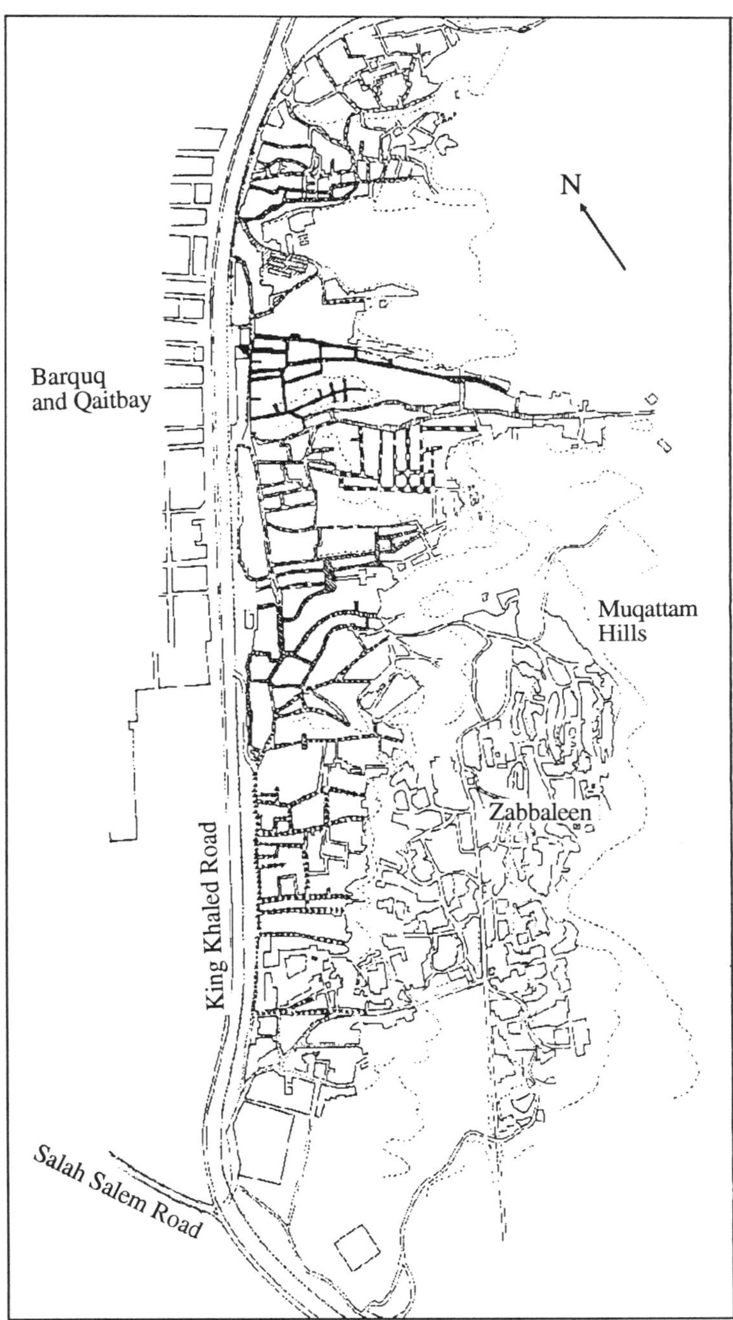

Figure 2-1. Garbage route map for Manshiet Nasser

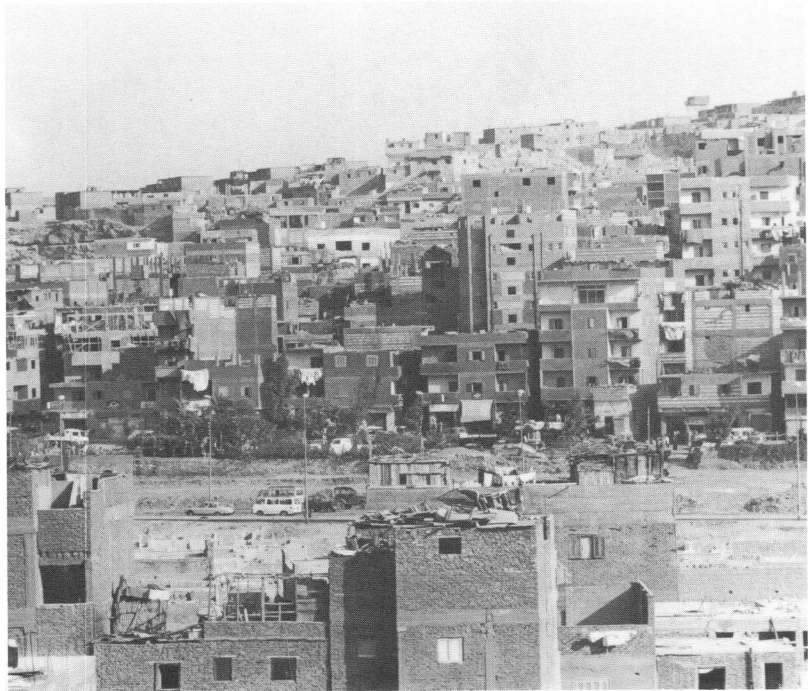

Manshiet Nasser

The garbage collectors serving Manshiet Nasser know its layout well. Their route map for the settlement, drawn in the early 1980s when they were preparing to offer collection services, is shown in Figure 2-1. Today, their donkey carts, and sometimes narrow vehicles, pass along the lanes shown in the map. The twenty-one routes, distinguished by different shadings of the lanes that lead upward to the interior, approximately define the areal extent of the settlement. When the present research was initiated, the expertise of these people helped us to map and divide the settlement into nine zones where the buildings and dwelling units were listed.

On the northeastern heights, Manshiet Nasser abuts another smaller settlement, Duweiqa, with no more delineation of the boundary than an internal roadway. Duweiqa is built on public land surrounding a large municipal dump. A heavy haze of smoke hangs over the Duweiqa settlement most of the time. This settlement contains multi-story government housing designed for evacuees from collapsed buildings in central Cairo, along with some privately constructed homes similar to those of Manshiet Nasser. There are also some flimsy structures, including tents, erected by families of nomadic origin.

While the hillside where Manshiet Nasser is located is public land and the inhabitants are legally squatters, the precariousness which this implies is not reflected in the physical structures of the settlement today. Most of the buildings are multi-storied, particularly at the older and lower elevations of the settlement, and are largely made of brick and reinforced concrete. There is nothing furtive or transient about the physical appearance of the individual houses which identifies them as illegal or temporary; it is only the relationship among buildings in terms of absence of air shafts and setbacks, and lengthy blocks without side streets, that suggests that this is not an officially planned community. Clearly the residents do not perceive eviction as an imminent danger.

The main entry to Manshiet Nasser is an unpaved road from the main highway about halfway along the length of the settlement. It crosses the rail track and becomes a road passing alongside the track inside the settlement. The first dwellings of the settlement were built near this entrance. There are other less important entries, each one sloping up from the highway and crossing over the railway to the dirt road that parallels the rail line on the Manshiet Nasser side of the tracks. We are calling this the 'spine road' of the settlement. A second road parallels the spine road inside Manshiet Nasser. This one is densely built up on both sides and has many commercial establishments. Lateral roads and lanes lead irregularly from the main interior road up into the slopes.

Manshiet Nasser has become a large, bustling community of houses, shops, and workshops, all co-existing without any pre-planned land-use configuration. In 1984, it accommodated over 64,000 residents and more than two thousand commercial and industrial establishments ranging from tiny grocery shops to aluminum foundries. It had a residential density of more than forty thousand persons per square kilometer, and was continuing to grow in density. About one-third of the population lives within two hundred meters of the spine road, where density is highest.

Neither Manshiet Nasser, nor any of the neighboring communities on the hilltops to the east or the flatlands and slopes to the north, existed prior to 1960. The settlement was founded in the early 1960s when a number of low income families living elsewhere in Cairo were evicted by urban building projects and needed a place to go. Prior to their move, the northern slopes of Muqattam were inhabited chiefly by fugitives from the law and by quarry guards. The area was barren rock graced by neither a water supply nor vegetation. The history of the Manshia, as residents refer to their community, is thus the history of a group, mostly quite poor, who managed to carve their living space out of an inhospitable environment. How they managed to establish a viable community on their own and made it grow is in itself a story worth knowing.

History of the Settlement

Origins

The nucleus of the Manshia community was formed by a group of families that was evicted from a self-help settlement located not far from the present site in a subdistrict of the Gamaliya (see map in Chapter 1). This community had grown near the historic bazaar area around the time of the Second World War. It was settled initially by migrants from Upper Egypt, predominantly from Qena and Sohag Governorates. A number of the migrants specialized in recycling low grade steel that they recovered from used oil drums. Over the years, people in this community developed a brisk trade in recovered steel. Others established warehouses on the site, and began to sell used building materials such as wood and bricks. The community of houses and warehouses that they constructed, mostly out of recovered steel sheeting, was called the 'sheet metal hamlet' ('Ezbat al-Safih). It was known throughout the city as a center for recycling and cheap supplies for the building trades. Construction workers, both skilled and unskilled, living in Upper Egypt or elsewhere in Cairo, came to join them seeking a place to live, to work, and to hire themselves out for jobs in the city.

The growth of the 'Ezba was one reflection of the profound changes that were occurring in the life of Cairo around the war years. The population of the city had increased strikingly during and immediately following the Second World War, as it did in cities all over the Arab world (Abu-Lughod, 1971:171–80; Issawi, 1982:102). Quartering of troops and shipping blockades raised demand sharply for locally produced goods. One elderly resident of Manshiet Nasser tells of working for the British army while he was living in the cemetery grounds, coincident with the founding of the 'Ezbat al-Safih settlement. Recycling of every useful material flourished, and the 'Ezba was built on this new industry.

Municipal authorities had warned the 'Ezba that construction of permanent shelters would not be tolerated at this location. An oft-recounted bit of the oral history of the settlement is the story of residents who hid permanent construction inside the temporary steel sheet walls to fool the authorities. By and large, however, the community was left undisturbed for many years. In about 1960, the Governorate of Cairo announced that it needed the land occupied by the 'Ezba to build a school and a hospital. Community leaders, including the one who functions as an *'umda* (local mayor or headman)[2] for the settlement, demanded that alternative living space be provided before eviction occurred. There ensued long negotiations which appear to have taken place over many months. The government was represented in these discussions by deputies of the National Assembly from the district in which 'Ezbat al-Safih was located. The authorities finally agreed that as 'compensation' they would arrange for tacit permission to be granted to the community to resettle on public land on the Muqattam hills. The elderly residents say the settlement was named Manshiet Nasser in honor of Egypt's president to help ensure continuing land tenure.

The designated place was in close proximity to the older parts of Cairo, but the land was then of little value. It was a rugged, inhospitable site with sharply diverging elevations, lacking all infrastructure, but the people agreed. The leaders were able to organize the move so that it could be carried out in a staggered way. Water was obtained from taps in mosques across the road in the cemetery of Qaitbay. Lighting was by kerosene lamps. The government provided three water taps along the main street of the community within a few months of the initial move.

Land development

The original settlers were concerned about security primarily because they did not have title to the land. They were also worried about the reputation of Muqattam as a refuge of criminals. They huddled together at the lower reaches of the hillside, building their houses on plots of land which were usually about 100 square meters, and their warehouses on larger plots. Some of the early settlers, however, staked claims to larger plots located farther up the hill, behind the initial cordon of houses, which were sold to newcomers later on.[3]

The leaders of 'Ezbat al-Safih, by then firmly established as the leaders of the new community, organized the division of land along the spine road near the main entrance. The divisions were made in a way which grouped people from the same areas of origin together. This arrangement was strengthened by families helping relatives and co-villagers to find space and settle near themselves.

Settlers recount a pattern of relatively rapid growth in the early years. Apparently every attempt was made to entice co-villagers and Cairenes of common origin from Upper Egypt to move to the settlement in the interests of mutual support and security. Once the front line of the settlement had been established, and perhaps even as it was being formed, a new pattern of land subdivision began to develop on the middle reaches of the steep hillsides. Families who came after the initial settlers would claim about two to three hundred square meters of land, build a home on approximately one hundred square meters and subsequently sell the rest to newcomers, usually relatives or people from their home villages. While the size of the plots may have been justified initially by hopes to build on all of the space, it turned out instead to be an effective mechanism for selecting one's neighbors. Plots were sold relatively inexpensively or sometimes simply given to relatives and co-villagers who could be depended upon for support in times of trouble and for cooperation in general.

Land continued to be freely available on the heights of the hillsides, beyond the settled area, for many years. At the lower levels, however, an informal but well-regulated system of validating claims on plots in the settled area came into existence. Persons would stake a new claim or purchase one from an earlier claimant. The land would not be considered definitively theirs unless they built on it within a reasonable period of time. In the interim between claiming and building, tenure was in question to a varying extent depending on the relationship of the claimant to the community as a whole, and to any other claimant in particular, and the location of the land itself.

The strongest claim to a plot was that of somebody already resident in the community who had no land or building. Such a claim was almost incontestable, and if contested the community would support the resident's claim against all others. The oral record of land transactions tells of a number of cases of persons who had claimed more than one piece of land, but were forced by social pressure to give up the second claim to persons who had no plot based on a sense of equity. It also tells of a case in the 1980s when the response to claim-jumping was murder.

The strength of a claim to land was somewhat weaker if a homeowner in the Manshia took the plot in order to build for children. Such a claim could be overridden by a family in greater immediate need, especially if the project was construction on behalf of a daughter; she is expected to take a husband who will provide housing for the couple after marriage. If a claimant was from outside the community and did not plan to take up residence soon after making a claim, that person would have difficulty sustaining the claim. The best course would be to erect a flimsy room on the plot and live there until permanent construction was started. Without the physical presence of the owner or, as a weaker choice, the immediate proximity of a close relative to act as a representative, the chances of being able to build would be low.

While the initial occupation of the settlement went forward without anyone's needing to pay for land, free land is no longer available. A market in land and buildings has emerged, because the supply is now limited relative to families wanting to settle in the community.[4] The residents are very much aware that they do not officially own the land. Therefore carefully worded bills of sale are written describing the money paid for a piece of land as money given to the original holder to 'leave it' to the buyer and not as the purchase price. In the case of built space, the building is described as personal property and the land as government owned.[5]

Sociopolitical organization

The growth of this community has been greatly influenced by the remarkable degree of internal sociopolitical order and cohesion it manifested from its early days. The community instituted a system of local governance and conflict resolution managed by a traditional headman (*'umda*) and supported by a council of elders, known as the 'Arab Council' (*maglis 'Arab*). This institution derives its model from the Bedouin system of governance, in which disputes are resolved within a hierarchical framework with the arbiter being the person or persons who constitute the link, at one level up, between the two parties. In the Bedouin model, a dispute between two brothers is resolved by their father, between cousins by their grandfathers, between more distant relations by the tribal elders, and between tribes by a council of elders. This model of conflict resolution was well-known to the elders of 'Ezbat al-Safih and subsequently Manshiet Nasser, as many of them, including the leader of the Council, originate from areas in Upper Egypt which have been strongly influenced by Arab traditions. Not themselves of Bedouin origin, they nonetheless succeeded in adapting this system in such a way that a highly flexible system of community governance emerged.

The council consists of a leader (*'umda*) and members who represent the areas of the country with the largest numbers of residents in the community. These are typically older men who have authority within their own particular segments of the community and who are known to the other segments. The residents who come from areas of the country with smaller numbers of residents may be associated with one of the larger groups, and their leaders are called to participate in deliberations when cases involving them are being discussed.

The council has functioned to contain and resolve disputes between individuals and families living within the area as well to represent community interests in relations with other communities and with public authorities. It has met nearly every day to resolve problems and disputes arising from diverse aspects of daily life in the community, ranging from family disagreements to disputes about land and housing, and commercial conflicts. In serious cases where formal authorities such as the police have to be involved, various cooperative arrangements are worked out, and conflict resolved as far as possible by the community itself. These typically allow the Council to reach some resolution of the dispute between the parties before formal procedures such as arrest are undertaken. Institutionalization of community interests within this type of a quasi-tribal framework has been important in enabling the community to manage the growth of the settlement in a relatively orderly manner and in obtaining modest amounts of resources from the official bureaucracy for the settlement. In the beginning the community's first concern was to minimize the attention of official administrative circles to the Manshia. Local dispute resolution and problem solving mechanisms made it possible to maintain a low profile.

As the community grew so did the need to adjudicate more and more conflicts. The need to interact with official bodies and to represent community interests also grew. Then came negotiations to increase urban services to the community. The penetration by government authority grew and the strength of the Arab Council ebbed, receiving a serious blow when the *'umda* himself died in 1989. As we shall see below, the sociopolitical framework has been steadily revised until a new structure could be said to have emerged by the early 1990s.

Economic history

The families who were involved in recovering and recycling sheet metal in 'Ezbat al-Safih continued to practice their trade in the workshops which they established in the Manshia. As the settlement grew in size and the threat of eviction receded, skilled workmen employed in workshops of the nearby bazaar area, making shoes, carpets and many other items, began to take advantage of the available land and open their own enterprises in the area behind the first settlers. The demand for construction workers grew as people moved into the settlement, making this an attractive location for reinforced concrete workers, masons, painters, electricians, plumbers, and carpenters serving both the settlement and the nearby neighborhoods of Cairo. By the early 1970s, coffee shops near the main interior road of the settlement were serving as recruiting stations where labor contractors would come from greater Cairo looking for skilled workers and day laborers. Up until the present, construction workers' coffee shops continue to be the key contact points for the construction labor market in Cairo. (Assaad, 1990b:20–22)

In the middle 1970s, international prices for copper rose so steeply that the traditional practice of providing the new bride with copper household utensils could not be sustained, and aluminum was substituted for copper on a wide scale. This change was facilitated by the establishment of a new aluminum smeltery in Upper Egypt (at Nag' Hammadi) using electric power from the recently completed Aswan High Dam. The old aluminum foundries which had depended on recycled and imported raw aluminum prior to the establishment of the Nag' Hammadi plant began to expand their production, and small workshops producing finished aluminum goods increased rapidly. The foundries constituted more and more of a nuisance in the densely populated Gamaliya area of Cairo where they were clustered. At about the time that the population at Manshiet Nasser was beginning to feel secure from eviction, municipal authorities began exerting heavy pressure on foundry owners to move out of the city center. Manshiet Nasser was an obvious alternative location, close to markets but with ample empty land and a low level of official attention. First one and then several foundries were established at the southern end of Manshiet Nasser, drawing in their wake many small aluminum workshops. As had been the case with the workshops founded during the early years, Manshiet Nasser offered land cheap enough for skilled workers to open their own establishments, and many of these workers-turned-entrepreneurs moved into the community as residents.

Just as the aluminum foundries and workshops had been sources of air pollution, noise, and unregulated work practices in the Gamaliya, so they became the same on an even larger scale in the Manshia. One indicator that the Manshia has become an officially recognized quarter is that the municipal authorities are once again in 1990 pressuring the foundries to move.

Portrait of Physical Growth in the 1980s

How housing is built and tenanted

A considerable stock of housing has been generated in Manshiet Nasser since the settlement began in the 1960s. The era of tin shacks and small independent structures is long past. Recently buildings of up to nine stories have appeared, showing that built space is reaching a high level of density. These buildings represent particularly substantial investments given the extremely irregular topography and steep slopes that characterize the location. Establishment of a surface sufficiently flat for building usually requires laborious leveling with hand tools and sometimes dynamite. Although land prices have been increasing steadily, it was still true in 1984 that the cost of leveling land for building often exceeded the cost of access to the land itself.[6] To make streets as settlement proceeds, the residents share the costs of leveling roads. In many cases they also share costs of cutting stairways into the hillsides for pedestrian traffic.

To finance construction, families show a remarkable ability to keep current household expenditures at a bare minimum in order to save every piaster. For loans, they draw not only upon their immediate family circle, but on more distant relatives and friends as well. Investment in housing is a very high priority for Egyptian families; to own a building which can house one's own family and those of one's children is the ambition of the great majority of Egyptian families.

When the self-help construction of a building gets under way, there are important inputs from the owner-builders themselves. They educate themselves in all aspects of construction and the building trades so that they will know how to finance, manage, and supervise every detail of the process. The owner–builder consults friends and kin who have themselves recently constructed or added to their homes concerning reliable tradesman, daily rates, relative advantages of payment by day or by piece, costs of materials, suppliers, alternate means of transport of materials, and various means of cutting corners. In short, the prospective builder turns himself into a serious contractor who devotes himself and family members unsparingly to the task. From the beginning, he usually lives in the community, as a previous renter or with friends, or he is building a better house to replace his present one, or for sons or daughters.

'Self-help' means that the owner-builder manages the construction process. If he is a construction worker by trade, or has relatives who are, the women and girls of the family will carry water for making mortar and wetting bricks. Recently, however, even men who are not in the construction trades, and occasionally women as well, are seen doing building maintenance or making improvements, saving on expenses by working themselves.

When the money is available to begin construction, an owner-builder takes time off from his work and together with his wife works closely with groups of skilled workmen, organizing and coordinating different stages of the construction. The owner-builder and his wife purchase all the materials, supervise workers, carry water (a construction input), and provide cigarettes, tea, and sometimes food for the workers. They may also help as support labor doing unskilled work such as carrying sand, bricks, and mortar. By building in stages, a room or a floor at a time, owners match the pace of construction with their ability to mobilize financial resources and their need for space. Buildings often take years to be completely finished.[7]

As soon as independent dwelling units are habitable—finishing work comes later—they are occupied by the owner's family or the newly marrying family members, or the units are rented. Shop rentals are also part of the economics of financing the cost of building. Space is seldom left empty. We found a vacancy rate for dwelling units of only 5 percent.[8]

The building stock is constantly expanded or improved as resources are accumulated. Since the first houses were built in the 1960s, construction has shifted from structures made solely of brick and cut rock to buildings framed with reinforced concrete and then filled with brick walls. There is a structural (not zoning) limit on height of two, at most three, floors, when the building is supported solely by brick or cut rock walls. Older buildings are razed and rebuilt with a reinforced concrete frame, reusing the original materials to fill in the walls. When floors are added, their design usually provides additional complete dwelling units rather than extra room space for existing units.

The tenants also participate in ongoing construction by providing demand for new units, renegotiating old rental agreements to pay for improvements, and also by engaging directly in improvements themselves with the permission of the owners. Most tenants prefer, wherever possible, to improve their units rather than move. A new rental normally requires a substantial upfront payment which is only partially offset by asking for a share in the 'key money' that the new tenant in one's old place will pay. These initial payments have risen rapidly with the inflation in housing costs and make a move very expensive indeed. Staying rather than moving is also preferred because access to valued goods and services, as well as ambiance and affective relationships, are tied to social networks which may take years to develop, and moves generally compromise them.

The case of one family illustrates the resourceful ways in which tenant families try to improve their housing space. A young couple with three children had been living in a single-room dwelling with a shared toilet in the building for LE 9.5 per month. After several years, a room across the hall became vacant. At that time, the family renegotiated the rental agreement with the owner to rent the other room, to be allowed to enclose the portion of the corridor between the two, and to build a toilet within part of this newly created private space. In return, they agreed to bear all the costs of the improvement and to increase the rent payment to LE 20 per month. A new official rent contract was drawn up with these provisions and the work carried out. By then the family consisted of 6 individuals, but they now had two rooms, hall space, and a private toilet of their own.

By the mid-1980s, a stock of approximately 14,000 dwelling units had been built. They were physically configured as shown in Table 2-1. The dwellings are organized most often in multi-floor buildings (60 percent), which is the trend as the settlement becomes more and more densely built. Another important configuration is a group of typically four to eight units (often single rooms) built around a small courtyard, sharing toilet facilities and a water tap, if any. This configuration (30 percent in 1984) remains only at the middle and higher (newly built) elevations and is declining in importance. Single dwelling units built as separate buildings have always been few; we found only 10 percent of this type. Many represent the first stage of housing capital accumulation and will be superseded later by larger multi-unit buildings.

Table 2-1. Physical characteristics of dwelling units

Living space	**Mean**
Rooms per unit (excluding toilet or separate kitchen)	1.85
By room size	**Percent**
One room	47
Two rooms	30
Three or more	23
All sizes	100
Facilities	
Separate kitchen (own use)	29
Own toilet	30
Sample Size N=1118	

Built space in the settlement is now bought, sold, and rented. However, title registration, building permits, regular enforcement of codes, and prior planning of physical layouts by the city are lacking. After two and a half decades of growth, Manshiet Nasser is no longer a settlement purely of self-help owners (Table 2-2). Our data show that 54 percent of the dwelling units were occupied by renters in the strictest sense of the term. If we add the families 'renting' from relatives, the figure is higher. Despite the high prevalence of renting, this is not an absentee-landlord community. Most owners of flats live in the same building or close by; they watch over their property carefully.

Rental is often a long-term arrangement that is the near equivalent of sale under the rent control laws. The owner retains control of shared space such as hallways, roof, and courtyard, and he controls all structural modifications. With the existing tenancy arrangements, all extensions of infrastructure involve complex negotiation and cooperation between tenants and owners. Rights of tenants, under rent control laws, are to a large extent observed, unless the parties make verbal agreements keeping open the possibility of subsequent renegotiation. A government-appointed housing committee, established under the rent control law, visits the settlement to review rents charged by owners and to set ceilings. Theoretically, renters can also obtain redress in the courts. This is expensive and takes a long time, so it does not happen often. However, a few cases have had a salutary effect by setting patterns for resolution of disputes outside the courts.

Table 2-2. Owners and renters of dwelling units

Occupant of dwelling unit	Percent
Owner (part or sole)	29
Renter from non-relative	54
Renter from relative	9
Rent free from relative	8
Where the owner of the dwelling unit lives	
Owner lives in own unit (owner-occupied)	29
Elsewhere in the same building	52
Elsewhere in settlement	10
Outside Manshiet Nasser	9
How owner acquired the dwelling unit	
Built	66
Bought	25
Inherited	9

Sample Size N = 1118

Table 2-3. Land use in the settlement

Plot use	Number of structures
Residential structures	
Exclusively residential	3,770
Structures that include shop space for commercial and manufacturing establishments (includes 2,093 shops and workshops)[a]	1,230
Structures committed exclusively to commercial and manufacturing use (266 establishments)[a]	159
Structures for social services	
Mosques	19
Schools	2
Health center[b]	1
Vacant plots	87
Under construction (use not yet defined)	212

a. The number of establishments given in parentheses totals 2,359. They are enterprises not plots, since there can be more than one shop or workshop in a building that occupies a single plot. The total number of establishments is subclassified into 1,504 shops and 855 workshops.

b. The health unit belongs to the Ministry of Health. It is located in a multi-story public housing structure that was built early in Manshiet Nasser's history for evacuees from other quarters of Cairo.

Source: Building survey, 1983.

Manshiet Nasser occupies a space of 1.5 square kilometers predominantly for residential use, though a significant amount of space is also used for commercial and industrial purposes (Table 2-3). The different uses of land are intermingled spatially and often occur in the same buildings, with residences above and commercial shops or workshops below. As we shall see in our discussion of economic production below, Manshiet Nasser is an attractive location for small enterprises. It has become an extension of the workshop areas historically located in a nearby quarter, the Gamaliya, which houses the old bazaar and many small businesses.

Regularization of tenure

This flourishing community of homes, shops, and workshops is in most respects legally invisible, though numerous links exist with public authorities for some services, and even for the application of rent control regulations. The granting of freehold tenure has been on the agenda since the late 1970s. This means that the costs of infrastructure (water, sewerage, roads, public buildings) installed under an upgrading program were to be distributed over the square meters of built land, with owners asked to purchase their land from the government at a price sufficient to pay for these installations. However, as of 1990 there had been no progress on this front. Officially this is because the city government wants to resolve land tenure issues citywide all in one action, rather than dealing with the communities included in upgrading programs one by one. Unofficially, the situation is that in the past thirteen years no one has ever been able to agree who can make the decisions about pricing of land in areas whose tenure is not recognized by the government, nor the mechanisms which will be used for legalizing. This whole issue is rife with rumors, ploys from the government, and counterploys from communities.

According to the conventional wisdom of urban area upgrading worldwide, the granting of secure legal titles to people who have in fact settled, but without permission, is supposed to galvanize their energies, causing them to convert from temporary to permanent housing, make home improvements, and become good citizens. The communities, once legalized, are also supposed to become more effective at establishing community institutions to solve problems that in their nature require joint, not individual solutions.[9]

The paradigm doesn't fit the upgrading sequence for Manshiet Nasser or other communities brought under upgrading projects during the late 1970s and 1980s in Cairo. People invested in permanent housing long before the upgrading projects were planned. The people could preempt the sequence because the government was not willing to raze the homes of residents unless they were severe nuisances. Thus, in such communities as Manshiet Nasser the settlement could reach a sufficient size of permanently housed residents to assure their security of tenure *de facto*, without need of the upgrading feature of freehold titles.

The community has also proceeded without benefit of legal tenure to face some of the problems that require joint action; e.g., the Arab Council brought 'law and order' relative to land claims and was able to settle family disputes and deal with some types of crime.

The most serious challenges, however, have arisen at the intersection of the community and Cairo's urban services, water and sewerage in particular. While housing can be built by individuals and small groups, whether legal or not, services from the city agencies that supply water, connect sewers, remove solid waste (garbage) from dumps, and pave roads, require recognition and cooperation from the official establishments. The question is, how does a community acquire these basic urban services when it exists actually, but does not exist in the legal framework surrounding the activities of the responsible government agencies. The answer in Egypt is that there is a polity and a long tradition of communities reaching into and mobilizing one or another government institution on their behalf. It has never been easy for people from the lower classes to do so, but they do have connections and networks through relatives and friends located at different levels of the vast bureaucracy. Often some help is obtained, and occasionally it is substantial, depending upon political and bargaining factors. Financial feasibility and the internal workings of each service organization differ, so each has to be approached uniquely.[10]

Organizing the infrastructure

The general situation in the mid-1980s was one of serious deficiencies in all urban services for the Manshia except two: electricity was connected throughout most of the settlement and a solid-waste (garbage) collection system for households was in place. All roads within the settlement area were unpaved and most were very narrow, frequently ending as blind alleys. The surfaces were uneven and gradients steep. For water connections and sewerage, the situation was also poor (Table 2-4).

The hilly topography and rock structure of the terrain raise the cost of placing pipes and pumps or siphons, which is a special problem in the Manshia not faced in most other settlements of Cairo. However, electric extensions could develop quickly, partly because the cost is less and collection of rates follows immediately. When illegal wires were strung, the end-users paid the owners at meter points. While this is illegal, and providers of electricity to neighbors risk confiscation of their electricity meters, this is temporary. The Electricity Authority provides meters to residents on demand, insisting only that owners meet the initial cost. The authority has a reputation for supplying services whether people have established a legal right of occupancy or not, whereas some of the other utility organizations have been much less forthcoming.

Sanitation and water are particularly important in this study because of their influence on health and illness, a subject which we discuss analytically in Chapter 5 below. For women and young girls, who must carry fresh water in and waste water out, these facilities make a great deal of difference. Costs are also raised when water is bought and waste must be removed by the householders. Manshiet Nasser's adaptation to the realities that had to be faced, and its progress toward better solutions will be discussed next. First, we take up sanitation, beginning with solid waste; then the system for

Table 2-4. Service connections

Service	Connected to dwelling unit	Elsewhere in building or courtyard
Electricity	90	na
Municipal sewer[a]	18	33
Municipal water tap	11	14
Sample size N=1118		

a. The survey did not assess whether the connection was working or not. We observed many that were blocked or improperly connected.

disposal of human waste and gray water. After that, we shall turn to the question of water requirements and how they are met in the Manshia.

During its first twenty years of existence, the Manshia had no household solid waste collection service. Street surfaces, vacant lots, and railway lines and other peripheral areas of the community were clogged with garbage placed there by residents who literally had no alternative. Children played in these areas, and residents had to pick their way around dumps when moving in and out of the community. In 1980, with the mediation of a private Egyptian organization, Environmental Quality International, a plan was agreed whereby the garbage collectors who live in the Zabbaleen settlement collect the household solid wastes of neighboring Manshiet Nasser on a regular basis in return for a monthly fee per household.[11] For one year the District Sanitation Department paid; thereafter the householders paid.

This venture became the occasion for the Zabbaleen to found their own private institution (*gama'iyya*) to take over management of the routes and fee collection. Ten years later, in 1991, the system continues to function well. The monthly fee has increased from LE 0.25 to LE 1.25 (now applying to groups of households in each building). The technology originally was donkey carts, but that too has changed. Small motorized vehicles that can negotiate the alleys now work alongside the reliable, even if dilapidated, donkey carts.

The collection service improved the cleanliness of the environment and increased awareness and commitment of the people to community sanitation. People appreciate the cleanliness and through social pressure have reduced the number of households throwing their garbage on dumps to a small number. Garbage continues to accumulate along the railway line, but it is dumped mainly by the market, shops, and workshops. Although the garbage collectors offer their service to these establishments for a fee, the temptation to dump rather than pay is there. Residents complain and the municipality periodically sends in trucks and crews to clear away the garbage on the community's perimeter.

Cairo had grown far beyond the capacity of its infrastructure by the time of the Second World War. The situation became progressively worse as the population more than doubled from its pre-war size up to the early 1970s. During the 1970s, massive foreign financial assistance became available, and a general strategy was adopted to solve accumulated problems of roads, water and sewerage. First, a large network of roads, flyovers and bridges was quickly built. Simultaneously, projects were initiated to dramatically increase the pumping capacity of the water and sewer networks and the length and size of their trunk lines. The new installations would carry the overloads already existing, and at a later stage the local networks themselves would be repaired and extended. According to this strategy, communities like Manshiet Nasser were last in line.

Fortunately, and despite many obstacles, there was one tenuous factor on Manshiet Nasser's side. A World Bank upgrading project for Egypt (see below) selected the community for special attention during the late 1970s. Through this exception to the general strategy, funding was made available to the government to install a local network within the settlement of sewers and water pipes. As we tell the story below, it took more than a decade and the project was neither completed nor up to engineering standards, but at the end there were some benefits for the community.

The principal technology for disposing of human waste in Manshiet Nasser is private pits cut out of the limestone rock in front of or alongside each building. These are rock vaults, not soak pits, so gray water (waste water) is introduced sparingly. The pits are emptied periodically. In 1984 this was done either by tanker vehicles with a pumping capacity or by laborers who carried the wastes out of the pits using buckets hung on shoulder poles. In both procedures, the sludge was carried only short distances before being dumped into empty spaces.

Since then, with increasing density and the development of small businesses in the settlement who offer cleaning as a service, a donkey cart system for pumping out the sludge is now used almost universally. By 1990 the service was available on call for an average fee per cleaning of LE 80, depending on terrain and size of the pit. Disposal is still on dumps, but at a further distance.

Many of the pits are connected to the sewage collection network, but we found many of these connections were not working properly in the mid-1980s. By 1990, the situation had improved after a decision by the parliament that the sewer organization should serve settlements being upgraded under programs funded by the World Bank or USAID. They responded by making an additional effort to extend the Manshiet Nasser network, but refused to make the individual connections, saying that these had not been specifically authorized. In consequence, many owners connected on their own, without official supervision. This may be a reason for the extensive leakage of sewage which spills onto the lower levels of the settlement, complicated by frequent breakages in the sub-standard mains. Spillage constitutes a serious risk of infection to anyone who lives on these streets, particularly children, who play in the roadways.

Without a second survey, we cannot specify the proportion of buildings now connected, but there has been an improvement over 1984 (see Table 2-4 above). Wherever there is piped water, there is now likely to be a sewer main as well. Earlier there was little coordination between the two systems except along the spine road at the bottom of the settlement. Many of the Manshia's water problems are connected with the sewer problem. One cannot use water in significant amounts unless there is a practical way to get rid of it afterwards.

Women in households lacking sewer connections typically dispose of domestic waste water, other than toilet wastes, by scattering it across the street surface. Neighbors insist that women do not dump their water at a single point, but sprinkle it around in the vicinity of the front door, to minimize the formation of ruts on street surfaces. Where the amount of water is limited, this is effective because evaporation is fast. As housing densities have increased, however, open ground has diminished, and the quantity of waste water which must be disposed of has increased, reducing the convenience of this system.

Obtaining sufficient water for drinking and other domestic uses is a major preoccupation of households in most self-help communities in Cairo. Communities established on the agricultural perimeters of Cairo use a variety of water sources when they cannot get municipal water: tubewells, canals, and the Nile itself. Manshiet Nasser, however, was built on the slopes of waterless hills, so all water for the community enters through municipal mains. Households lacking connections with the water system mostly obtain their water from other households which have connections, though some take from public taps.

Water mains were installed first along the lower reaches of the settlement. While this would have been quickly followed in most communities by a proliferation of self-help water connections, there was not enough water pressure to carry the water up the hillsides of Manshiet Nasser. At the time of the survey, one-quarter of the households of the settlement had piped water inside their dwelling units or elsewhere in their buildings (Table 2-4 above). Even for these households, the city-wide problem of irregular and insufficient pumping pressure meant frequent cuts or no water at all. On an individual basis, some of the more affluent residents have installed private household pumps that lift water to tanks placed on the roof. This helps some people, but empties the mains and induces others to follow suit in a self-defeating competition.

Household members, particularly women, allocate considerable time and often money to the acquisition of water. Most households have intricate arrangements to ensure an adequate water supply. They use more than one source: their own taps, taps of households which sell water, public taps (whose water is carried by women of the household or by someone else for a fee), and delivery carts. Even for those with piped water, low pressure and cuts in service are frequent enough that households need to supplement from

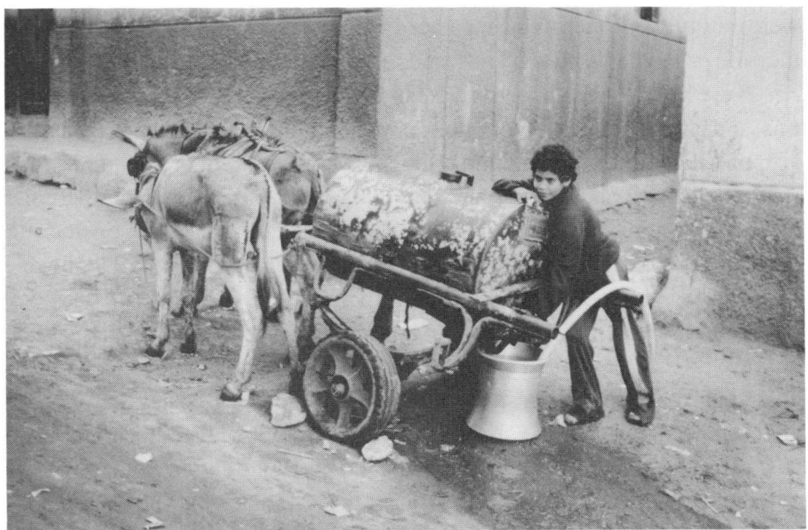

Home delivery of water. Photograph by Nadir Hashem.

other sources and to store water. The most prevalent alternative to one's own tap is the tap of someone else. Public taps play only a minor direct role in supplying domestic water, though they are used by delivery carts as a source.

From dawn to dusk there are long lines of women and young girls patiently waiting their turn to draw water in front of buildings along the main street. One woman recounted breastfeeding the child of a woman whose own milk supply had failed, as an act of kindness and charity, but also, as she laughingly reported, 'It is convenient and good insurance to have access to her water tap.'

It is mostly the women and young girls who provide their households with water. Training in water-carrying is an important part of preparation for womanhood. Mothers start their daughters at an early age, teaching them to carry water in a small metal container (*bastilla banati*—girl's container) balanced on their heads. When one or more teenage daughters or daughters-in-law are available to carry water, the mother phases herself out of water carrying. Whenever possible, pregnant and lactating women are exempted from water carrying, but in young families without others to help or that cannot afford to pay someone to carry or deliver water, these women also have to carry.

Everyone has to have a water carrying system. Women and young girls may help fetch water for male relatives living alone, elderly kin, or families of young men to whom they are engaged. Women may carry water for payment for men living alone. Occasionally men carry water. About 6 percent of the households that carry their water mentioned male members as carriers. They were mostly single men living together, or men whose wives were away. Where the wife or mother is present, husbands and sons rarely carry water.

Every home, whether it has a tap or not, stores water in an array of pots, tins, and barrels. The most common container is the barrel (*barmil*), the larger size of which holds three hundred liters. Over 40 percent of the households had at least one such barrel and one household had seven. Total storage capacity is highly variable, averaging 270 liters per household. Considering the small size of most dwelling units in this settlement (see Table 2-1 above), water storage consumes a good deal of living space.

Water is also a high cost input to household life in Manshiet Nasser. The energy and time of women and girls is a cost even if undervalued, containers cost money, and the living space allocated to storage is a cost. Finally, there are current expenses to pay for water. The magnitude of the time and energy cost is broadly suggested by the fact that 64 percent of households carry all of their water, and another 17 percent carry at least some of it. Only about one-fourth of households obtain water without carrying, by taking it from taps in their own homes or buildings, or from donkey cart vendors. The dependence upon carrying where the terrain is difficult and there are long lines at taps reflects the tight income constraints under which people live.

That was the situation in the mid-1980s. The basic patterns remain, but two important improvements were seen by the early 1990s. First, a pumping station with a large storage tank has been built at the Citadel end of the settlement on the highest point. This was part of the agenda of the World Bank project, so long delayed in implementation. The mains have been extended and feed the system below. It seems that this system is working well. It does not serve the entire settlement, because some areas are at too high an elevation or pipes were not placed for the local area. We estimate, without benefit of a survey, that more than half of the households now have piped water. Some parts of the settlement, however, still have no running water at all, not even standpipes.

The second important improvement is the development of a more standardized and economical system of private water delivery. Now there are small vehicles plying the narrow streets selling water in standard containers. They are everywhere, supplementing the supply from small tank trucks that are pulled by donkeys. With water cuts still frequent, and many homes without water, these systems of home delivery are vital. Water continues to be carried and hosed from dwelling to dwelling, but not to the extent of earlier years. The water is sold in returnable containers,[12] each with fifty liters of water. A deposit is paid and the containers are rotated when a filled one is purchased. The price is LE 0.35 at the higher elevations and LE 0.15 lower down. This is small-scale private business filling a major gap not tended by the public services. It is headquartered on the spine road at the bottom where water supply is best.

The present system is more cost-effective for the residents than the choices available in 1984. At that time, we found that households that were buying water spent an average of LE 4.20 per month It is now cheaper, in real terms, and there are fewer women and girls carrying water. On the assumption that households must replenish their supply of stored water on a five-day cycle, the monthly cost for those who cannot refill from taps in their own buildings is about LE 8.10 per month in 1990.[13] The international value of the Egyptian pound has meanwhile decreased to one-third what it was at the earlier date.

The World Bank 'up-grading' project

International lending and aid agencies came to Egypt in the mid-1970s on a wave of international studies—mostly in Latin America—of so-called squatter or informal urban settlement, each with suggestions about what should be done to channel and build upon the inherent energy of the new settlements. The World Bank joined with the Egyptian government to pursue what came to be known as the Egypt Urban Development Project, funded and technically advised by the Bank. This project included components for the upgrading of Manshiet Nasser's physical infrastructure, and provision of health, educational and social facilities. The plan was to regularize tenure by selling the land to building owners at a square-meter price sufficient to cover the costs of the infrastructure. Regularization of tenure has not been achieved, but some of the physical aims were partially or wholly realized.[14]

The project commenced in 1977, but then had to be stretched out, finally ending with its official closure in 1985. We saw some of the sewerage and water distribution systems in place at the time of our survey. The pumping station, school, and social buildings were completed later by Egyptian organizations that followed through after the project had been officially closed.

While all this was going on, there was a public debate and many meetings on whether 'informal' settlements should be bulldozed or assisted. In practice, the bulldozer approach was rarely used, and only when small numbers of squatters settled in defiance of other building plans. Public money for housing typically went to build housing for public employees, or for people evicted when public space was needed, or whose houses had collapsed—needy groups. Some public housing was built in Duweiqa, next to Manshiet Nasser, to house families who were relocated.

The World Bank project was relevant to this debate because it tried to show that public money could also be used to support the self-help community building process. This approach is demonstrably cheaper than public housing and it responds directly to demand. The idea that tenure could be regularized with title deeds in exchange for assessments on improvements never worked out. It is a moot point whether a system of assessments could ever have been agreed that would speed up the extension of infrastructure which is what the residents want. They are not worried about eviction. Yet it is obvious that capital projects such as pumping stations and trunk lines for sewers and water can only be organized under a public authority, which takes money and time; the complaint is that it takes too much time.

Portrait of Social Conditions in the 1980s

Who lives here: regional and local origins

This particular settlement has a strong infusion of Upper Egyptian backgrounds, which is the origin of much of Cairo's outborn population. The Manshia's household heads were born mainly in Asyut, Sohag, and Qena in Upper Egypt. Fayoum, which is an hour's drive to the southwest of Cairo, was also the birthplace for many residents. Nevertheless, the majority of household heads (61 percent) moved to Manshiet Nasser from Cairo, some of them as native-born Cairenes and others as second-stage migrants from Upper Egypt.

First-generation Upper Egyptians are still the dominant group among property owners in the Manshia. Their lifestyles, political alliances, and ideas have dominated the life of the settlement since the outset. However, this generation is becoming elderly, and many of the founding residents, including the *'umda* himself, have died. As the children of the Manshia themselves have matured, the customs and values that they have learned at the social

Table 2-5. Origins of household heads: percentages by place of birth and last residence prior to Manshiet Nasser

Regional origins	Place of birth	Last residence prior to Manshiet Nasser
Cairo[a]	31.6	60.6
Upper Egypt, mainly Assiut, Sohag, Qena	46.2	26.4
Fayoum[b]	11.3	7.3
Lower Egypt (Delta)	9.3	4.0
Canal and frontier	0.4	1.0
Manshiet Nasser	1.2	0.6
All	100.	100.
Sample size N = 1118		

a. Respondents from places nearby in Giza or Qalyubia could not always tell us clearly whether they came from our definition of metropolitan Cairo or not, so we think there is some overstatement of Cairo origins.

b. Fayoum is a fertile depression in the desert one hour's drive southwest of Cairo. Officially it is classified as part of Upper Egypt.

intersections of the settlement and the city have become stronger factors. The hold of provincial custom is likely to be loosened, and that very special Cairo distillate, expressed as the *baladi* living style, may weaken; at the very least it will be modified.

To be *baladi* is to identify oneself as having a lifestyle that preserves many of the values concerning dress, honor, marriage, honesty, and extended family relationships of Upper Egyptian life (seldom are these people Delta migrants). The women are conspicuous by their wearing of ankle-length black wraps, the *milaya-laff* or the *abaya*, with adequate display of contour and movement to be attractive. *Baladi* is an urban, not rural, lifestyle. Such families live mostly in nuclear households, men rule, but women are strong, and the airs of the 'modernized' middle and upper urban classes are eschewed. A person can be accepted from the higher classes as *baladi* if they hold to the same personal standards and acknowledge their own solidarity with this sub-cultural group, but this is exceptional (el-Messiri, 1978:522–40).

The current stream of in-migrants is households predominantly formed by young couples, two-thirds of whom had moved to the community from elsewhere in Cairo. Some had already started their families (a little less than half of the couples), probably while living briefly as newlyweds in their parental homes; others came to the community as couples without children, presumably with plans to start their families in Manshiet Nasser.

While three-fourths of the migrant households were young families, the other one-fourth was an assortment of generally non-family households. They were formed mostly of males, workers and students, and came largely from outside Cairo, i.e. they were truly new migrants to Cairo and settled first in Manshiet Nasser, typically renting one-room dwelling units.

Demographic factors

The population of Manshiet Nasser reached 64,000 by the mid-1980s, large enough to have its own internal growth dynamics on top of the contribution of continuous in-migration. Natural increase alone (births minus deaths) was raising the population at a rate of 3.5 percent per year. When in-migration is added, the rate of increase was running at not less than 5 or 6 percent per year. We could not measure the rate of in-migration precisely, but reasonably good estimates of the other demographic parameters could be made (Table 2-6). To put them in context, rates for metropolitan Cairo are also shown, referring to approximately the same date. Since both fertility and mortality are falling continuously in Cairo, dating is important whenever demographic rates are compared.

Manshiet Nasser's demographic rates are more like the averages for Upper Egypt than the averages for Cairo. However, this can be deceptive. If

Table 2-6. Measures of fertility and mortality for Manshiet Nasser and metropolitan Cairo: dates around 1984

Demographic measure	Manshiet Nasser	Metropolitan Cairo
Total fertility per woman[a]	5.3	3.7
Contraceptive prevalence (percent of married women under age 50 currently using contraception)	18.8	45[d]
Infant mortality rate (deaths per 1000 births)[b]	110	73
Expectation of life at birth in years for both sexes combined[c]	52	62

a. The total fertility rate is total births over the life course given current age-specific birth rates with no deduction of births for women who die before reaching the end of their reproductive period. The particular structure of age and marital status in Manshiet Nasser imparts an upward measurement bias for which an adjustment has been made.

b. Infant and child mortality is measured for Manshiet Nasser by the indirect 'Brass' method, and for Cairo by vital registration data with a small adjustment for omissions (see chapter 4 below). Technical precautions were taken to avoid measurement biases due to in-migration.

c. The expectation of life is an approximation based on measurements of child mortality (see note b) which are then extrapolated for the rest of life by 'West' model life tables.

d. An estimate for urban Egypt from the 1984 Contraceptive Prevalence Survey.

Sources: Present study; for metropolitan Cairo see Shorter (1989)

people of the same class in Cairo are compared with Manshiet Nasser, the differences would be much less, or might disappear altogether. This point is discussed in relation to infant mortality in Chapter 4 below.

With respect to fertility, a significant comparison is reproductive behavior; contraceptive prevalence was 19 percent in the Manshia while it was 17 percent for a similar date in Upper Egypt and 45 percent in Cairo as a whole—again without benefit of data by comparable classes in Cairo.[15] We do not take this to mean that the Manshia is a simple transplant from Upper Egypt, because there are secular changes going on in both places. The general averages for contraceptive prevalence are rising in Upper Egypt as they are in Cairo. The young families of the Manshia are slightly ahead of the path of change seen as averages for Upper Egypt, again without adequate information on class-specific behavior.

It must be stressed that these data are all for dates around 1984, and the situation is changing rapidly. Between 1984 and 1991—only seven years—a comparison of contraceptive prevalence rates from two national surveys shows an increase from 30.3 percent to 47.6 percent in the country as a whole.[16] For every two women who were contracepting in 1984, more than three were doing so by 1991. Total fertility has been falling correspondingly.

While we cannot assign a similar path of change mechanically to the Manshia, some such increase is highly probable, because the general trend has been confirmed by measurements in all regions of Egypt, including both rural and urban settlements.

Meanwhile, the population of Manshiet Nasser is being built by natural increase and in-migration both. To get a clearer idea of the dynamics of the settlement's growth, we shall focus on households, not individuals, since it is the formation of new households, not the bearing of babies as such, that puts pressure on the market for dwelling units.

One source of new households is young families, often newly-married, who move to Manshiet Nasser to make their homes. Once settled, they build their families. For quite a while, until their children reach marriageable ages, there is no further demand from them or their progeny for dwelling units; although they may modify their own unit to add rooms. Eventually, however, the children grow up, marriages need to be arranged, and thus a fresh demand for space arises. It must be found either in Manshiet Nasser or by spilling out to other affordable places.

Manshiet Nasser is different from the general averages of Cairo in the importance of young families. This can be seen in the age structure of women from age twenty onwards (Figure 2-2).[17] We look at women because they are responsible for childbearing and without them there are no families. In Manshiet Nasser the women are distinctly young and building their families. Their unmarried 'sisters' are living in Cairo or Upper Egypt where they will stay until they are married, so they don't get into the curve for Manshiet Nasser. When they do marry they will think of moving from the parental home to Manshiet Nasser or another affordable place.

Figure 2-2. Female population above age 20: Manshiet Nasser and Cairo, 1985

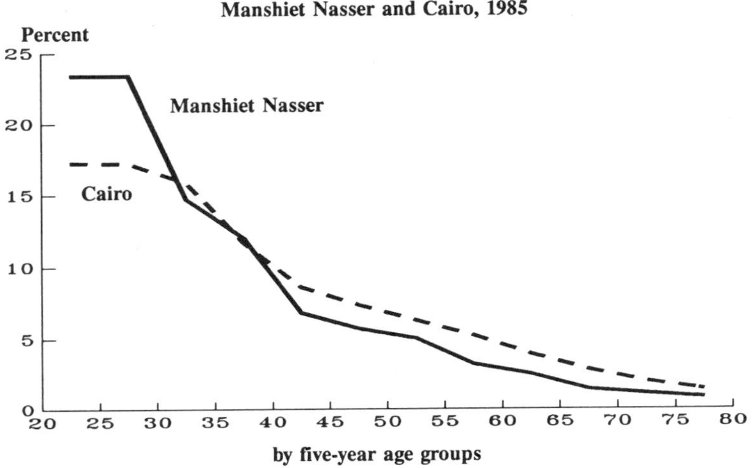

Figure 2-3. Projected increase of female population by age: 1985–2010 (excluding migration)

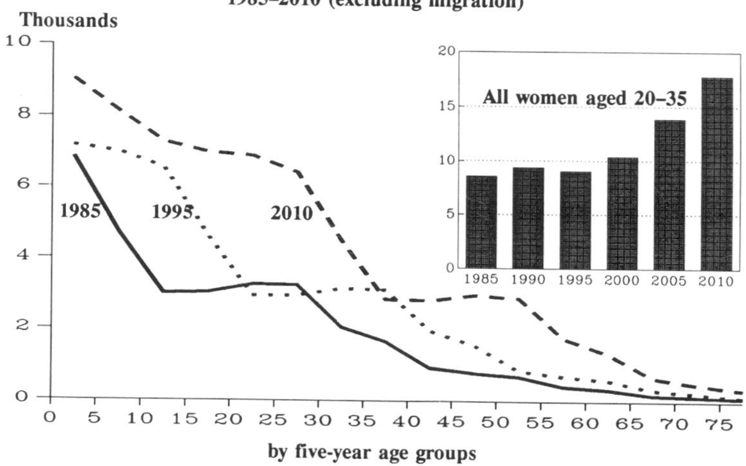

Continuing this line of thinking, we may look at the entire age range of females as it was in 1985 and as it will develop in the future for the women who were already residents in 1985, i.e. as a result of natural increase alone. The process is shown by making a population projection from 1985 as in Figure 2-3.[18] The steep left-hand portion of the curve for 1985 shows the result of high childbearing in the recent past. There is also a concentration of women around ages twenty to thirty, virtually all of them married and most of them have recently moved into Manshiet Nasser. The age-selectivity of their moves to Manshiet Nasser creates an irregularity in the curve. That same hump is seen in the curves for 1995 and 2010, but shifted to the right (to higher ages), because the selected group of women becomes older as each of these later dates is reached.

The original group of women (1985) have their children during their twenties and early thirties. The children grow up, and a second bulge appears echoing the first one. The second one is seen in the curve for the year 2010 (look at ages twenty to thirty) when they, in their turn, become mothers. There are more women in 2010 than in 1985 due to the more-than-replacement reproduction that has taken place. The bar diagram shows how the increase in numbers of young adult women, slow at first, becomes rapid. Almost every one of these women will marry and need housing.

In time, there will be a great increase in demand for housing in Manshiet Nasser, on top of what we have been seeing in the past, stemming solely from natural increase. It will have to be met from within the settlement, or by young people moving out to find affordable housing elsewhere—or delaying their marriages for a while. Thus, we can predict with near certainty that within five or ten years following publication of this book, another boom in demand for housing, on top of all the rest, will be felt in Manshiet Nasser.

Summarizing this complex, but important, line of reasoning, there are two waves of increase in the population that bring increases in the demand for housing. One occurs at the time cohorts of young adults move into the settlement as migrants. These migrants are the source of a second wave of housing demand that is initiated by having births, which, after a time lag, lead to the formation of young families that need places to live. All the while, both waves are generating more population in Manshiet Nasser, offset slightly by deaths. Thus, even if economic forces brought in-migration to a halt, there would be more growth in store for Manshiet Nasser by the momentum of natural increase alone.

There are other, lesser forces building the size of the community: workers come to the settlement to find temporary quarters, and then there are students from the provinces who have come to Cairo for education. Occasionally, older people come to the settlement to be near close relatives such as their children, or friends, or they come for economic reasons. Housing is not cheap in Manshiet Nasser, but it is cheaper than some of the alternatives.

The limits to growth of Manshiet Nasser are much more likely to be due to economic factors than to a slowing down of demographic reproduction, even though that may also happen. Costs of adding floors to buildings, and then demolishing buildings to make way for structurally sound high-rise buildings, all add up to more expensive housing. People who look for housing, including young couples who grow up in Manshiet Nasser, will compare affordability with housing elsewhere on the perimeters of Cairo, balancing cost differentials against the loss of daily access to social support systems in the community entailed by a move.

When looking to the future, the increase of households in the Manshia is likely to be constrained by economic factors, forcing some of the demographic momentum to spill over into other parts of Cairo. Our demographic projection, without in-migration, for natural increase alone, gives a population of 105,000 by the year 2000 and 135,000 by the year 2010. However, one ought to add to these figures the effect of in-migration which is continuing. This causes one to wonder what the ultimate limits to this community are. Surely, costs and affordability will prevent such high densities from materializing—or will they? If medium-rise buildings of ten or so stories become the rule, then it could happen.

Social infrastructure

By social infrastructure, one means the systems that people draw upon for educational and health services, for assistance in times of exceptional need, and the sociopolitical organizational structures of the community. Part of the infrastructure of a community is governmental, and part consists of private institutions of the civil society. Thus, the general structure includes private voluntary organizations (secular or religious), private professional practitioners (physicians, healers, midwives, tutors), and businesses (pharmacies, commercial schools). Also of great importance are social networks built on various bases, formed principally of relatives, neighbors, and workplace friends.

As the demand for social services grew with the settlement's own expansion, private social services were the first to materialize. They kept pace remarkably well with the growing demand. State services were much slower to be established within the settlement. Some services, such as hospitals and schools, were accessed by going outside Manshiet Nasser to neighboring parts of the city. As each type of social infrastructure is discussed below, the inherently greater flexibility of private voluntary and business institutions in responding to community needs is apparent.

For the government, new settlements such as Manshiet Nasser are financial and administrative 'inconveniences' in a city that is both short of resources for this purpose and strapped down by its own bureaucratic policies and procedures. In the long run, both private and public structures are necessary for the full development of the community. The complaint has

Coming home from school. Photograph by Nadir Hashem.

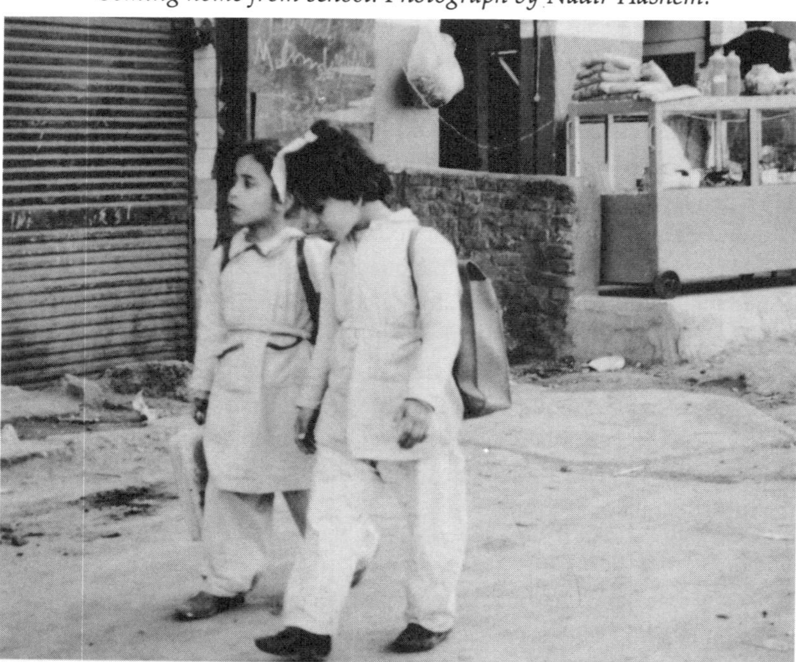

consistently been that the public services are very slow to materialize, even after the relevant service provider organizations accept the demands as proper ones in principle.

Schools

In 1984 there were more than nine thousand children of primary school age in Manshiet Nasser, but only two small primary schools. Our survey showed that 69 percent of boys and 56 percent of girls eligible to attend primary school were doing so (1984). Comparable figures for Cairo as a whole are 96 and 95 percent respectively (1988). Almost all of the Manshia's children had to walk considerable distances to other districts across the railroad tracks, highway, and cemeteries.

Since the relevance of formal schooling tends to vary by social class, the differences might be a little less if the Cairo standard of comparison were for children of the same class as Manshiet Nasser. Girls are relied upon for home chores, and it is only recently that formal schooling has begun to enter the parents' calculus of how best to prepare them for marriage and adult life. A deterrent for boys is that some have started to contribute to family income or are learning trades; seven percent of boys in the Manshia of primary school age were reported to be working as apprentices in workshops or in the construction trades.

By the year 2000 there will be, on account of natural increase alone, seventeen thousand children of primary school age. If all children can attend primary school by then, the stream of graduates eligible for entry to secondary school will be an additional challenge.

Yet access to schooling is improving in the Manshia. By 1990, four more primary schools had been built. Student capacity had reached about 7,500 with double shifts.[20] One of the new schools is the el-Gabarti Primary School at the top of the hill on the border between Manshiet Nasser and the Zabbaleen settlement. A three-year preparatory school was built on the same site, opening in 1989. One could say that this was an average rate of progress for educational facilities in a new community in Cairo, reflecting the way that social infrastructure follows rather than accompanies trends in basic needs.

Suzanne Mubarak, the wife of Egypt's President, took a special interest in the Manshia and Zabbaleen communities. This encouraged both private voluntary organizations and government ministries to strengthen their efforts on behalf of the Manshia.[21] An important contribution was also made by staff of the World Bank project who followed the el-Gabarti School and social affairs complex through to completion, overcoming a number of serious construction problems.

Many children from the Manshia continue to walk to primary schools in Duweiqa, Barquq, and Qaitbay; and some children from those quarters travel the reverse route to attend the schools in Manshiet Nasser. One now sees many children in their school uniforms on the dirt lanes of the community, walking back and forth to school as each shift takes its turn. While primary schooling is improving in coverage, only one school offers students the opportunity to continue through the middle school level. Though we saw some indications in 1984, there were many more signs in 1990 that parents were viewing schooling for girls as well as boys as useful preparation for work and marriage. The data from the survey show that higher proportions of the younger children are in primary school than was the case with the older ones who went before them. Furthermore, continuation rates above the primary level are also increasing.

There are other educational programs in the community. These include courses in sewing provided by private voluntary organizations with support from the Ministry of Social Affairs. Many children, mostly boys, attend Quran schools as well as primary school. Significantly, there are also twelve typing schools for girls of secondary school age in Manshiet Nasser, clearly an indication of a desire to prepare daughters for white-collar employment.

Nursery schools have begun to multiply. Informal custodial arrangements among neighbors have always been there, but organized care with educational objectives was not widely available at the time of the survey. The nursery schools are being established by private voluntary organizations, mosques, and private organizations. Five private nursery schools charge between LE 5 and LE 8 per month. The schools are being patronized because parents in this community are placing a higher value on education, not because larger numbers of women are going to work. Parents see nursery school as a head start on primary school.

Health care facilities

In 1984, there was a single government health unit that served few people, but then people obtain much of their medical care from private not government sources in Egypt. Families depended upon private clinics that opened evenings in the settlement, or they went to out-patient services of the government hospitals elsewhere in the city. Yet at that time 2,900 Manshia mothers were delivering babies each year, infants who would need medical care from time to time. Projections show that the number of deliveries by women who are already living in the Manshia (not including additional migrants) will rise to 3,400 by the year 2000.[22]

At the beginning of the 1990s, the original public health unit had been reactivated for use as a medical staff training facility; it has more than seventy doctors working there at a time. It also has an ambulance. The unit is open for public service only in the mornings, and people complain that the ambulance is often unavailable after hours. With wry Egyptian humor, it is said that illnesses and accidents should behave better, and keep government hours like everyone else.

Private clinics have multiplied; a reasonable estimate is in excess of one hundred. Five groups of private doctors have established polyclinics that are open twenty-four hours a day and their business is booming. The private medical profession has certainly responded to the demands of an increasing population in Manshiet Nasser. The profession as a whole in Egypt is suffering from an oversupply of physicians trained by the numerous medical schools. This helps to explain the quick professional response to community demand.

Private voluntary organizations

In the mid-1980s, private voluntary organizations in the Manshia were mainly associations based on region of origin. In addition to these, the Ministry of Social Affairs had established the Manshiet Nasser Community Development Association which carried out a few limited community services. The Ashira el-Mohamadia Association, which is an Islamic private voluntary organization with private external funding, operated a multi-purpose outpatient clinic, a small in-patient clinic, an evening sewing training center, and a day care center. Its activities, however, were restricted to a small part of the settlement.

A newly-formed Association for the Development and Enhancement of Women, based outside the settlement, started an income-generating project for female-headed households in both the Zabbaleen and Manshiet Nasser communities as their first undertaking in 1986. It is continuing and works mainly with older women who have no male wage income, usually due to widowhood or divorce, but sometimes due to disability or unemployment of the husbands. Small loans for production activities are given. These households are female-headed in the sense that their sole or primary economic support comes from a woman. The designation of headship in other respects is universally male, to the extent of naming relatives who may not even live in the household. As a social classification, identification of the breadwinner serves better for some purposes.[23]

There were eight community organizations—Muslim, Christian, and secular—in Manshiet Nasser in 1990. All of them have nursery schools or plan to open one (see above on schools.) Other activities are sewing classes for girls, literacy training, medical clinics, women's clubs, and tutoring. The two largest and best funded are the Islamic associations, which draw a substantial part of their funding from abroad. One of these is setting up a chain of nursery schools around the community.

In addition, the large number of associations based on community of origin that were present at the time of the initial survey are still active in 1990. Their programs are mostly restricted to burials, Quran memorization, and sometimes small emergency loans, but they also play a role in dissemination of news of regional interest.

At the new social services complex at the top of the hill (adjacent to the el-Gabarti school), a Cairo-based private voluntary organization, the Integrated Care Society for Primary School Children, provides staff and supervises health care services for children and their mothers. The Society works together with the Ministry of Health so that some government supplies, equipment, and government staff are also brought into the center. The patient load is about three thousand per month.[24]

In addition to privately organized services, a social affairs unit of the Ministry of Social Affairs is present in Manshiet Nasser. It undertakes a variety of activities, including the supervision of nursery schools and the community-level administration of the Egyptian government's pension system. Pensions are given to divorcees, widows, orphans, disabled persons, the elderly, spinsters, and the wives of draftees. The amount of money is small, usually no more than LE 10 per month. The state system reflects the social value that material assistance and sympathy should be offered, because these people are deemed to be needy through no fault of their own. However, what is achieved through these state programs is pitifully inadequate.

Sociopolitical organization

The Arab Council discussed above does not have the influence today that it had in the early years of the settlement. Weakening of its influence could be seen as the community was being drawn into the web or formal institutions through establishment of such facilities as a police station and an office of the leading political party. The death of the *'umda*, who had guided and protected the settlement since its days at 'Ezbat al-Safih, and who had a real genius at maintenance of community support and control functions, dealt the system a blow from which it could not recover.

This system would have died in the end in any event, however. The circumstances under which younger men have been raised, and the environment in which they must work out their own ambitions are quite different than those for the elders of 'Ezbat al-Safih; many of them never lived in Upper Egypt, and even those born in 'Ezbat al-Safih were never leaders there because they were too young. They rarely have the personal skills needed to adjudicate disputes or to establish community consensus. The Council still meets, but not nearly as often, and although those who are building local political careers along these lines say it is as powerful as ever, they don't agree on who is important. Their voices do not carry conviction when they discuss the salience of the Arab Council.

Meanwhile, the citizens of Manshiet Nasser no longer have the same incentive to keep a low profile, nor can they, as was good strategy during the community's early years. The Manshia's existence today is a *fait accompli*, recognized by the municipal administration. There is now a police station, established for a newly-delineated administrative district (*qism*) and its seven sub-districts (*shiakat*). Included are the cemeteries of Qaitbay and Barquq as well as neighboring settlements such as the Zabbaleen.

When we refer to Manshiet Nasser, we mean the historical delineation that local people recognize, which is sometimes called the main settlement of Manshiet Nasser. As it is integrated into the urban system, it loses some of its distinctive flavor and independence in exchange for legitimacy as a Cairo community. This in turn means that it can negotiate for official services, and its citizens can participate more effectively in city and national politics. Thus, there is now opportunity for ambitious young people to rise to leadership through official channels, such as the formal political party system, but less opportunity for charismatic leaders from within the community to take independent charge of local events as happened earlier through the Arab Council.

Social Networks

In the city, as in the countryside, individuals and households are connected to other individuals and households, as well as to institutions, by a web of personal relationships. For newcomers to the Manshia, the organizing principles of these relationships are initially those of kinship or place of origin, which may include friends made in other Cairo neighborhoods. Over time these networks expand to include neighbors and colleagues, such as co-workers of men or women who travel outside the settlement, in an ever expanding web.

For women more than men, but even for men, residential proximity is important in the formation of networks. They retain relationships, especially those of kin, that pre-existed in distant parts of the city, but travel is necessary and not always convenient. The spatial configuration of urban life consequently forces atrophy of some networks and the development of others. As time has passed and the community has matured, however, there has been a major increase in the reach and complexity of networks for both men and women.

Social networks of the Manshia mediate access to many kinds of resources, including material goods and services, information, and emotional support. Individuals rely on networks of reciprocal exchange to find employment, ensure job security, obtain interest free loans of cash, buy or build housing, and facilitate routine tasks by borrowing food, clothing, labor, and small household items. These networks also constitute the context within which beliefs, attitudes, and practices, including ones which foster child health, are formulated and changed. Exchanges promote security, cooperation, and trust among community residents. Reciprocity is implicit and weaves bonds of trust supported by kinship, common origin, neighborliness or collegiality.

Networks are used by Manshia residents to gain entry to public distribution systems in health, education, and subsidized goods. Such networks enable otherwise powerless people to manipulate redistribution systems of the state for their own benefit. These personalized systems also enable residents to gain control over preferential market transactions which are rife in the market economy.[25]

Women's networks

Myriad tiny grocery stores dot the streets of the settlement, and they have become the sites for social interaction among women. Public taps are at a distance and women mostly buy from water trucks anyway. Laundry is done inside the houses. Women rarely if ever visit the homes of non-relatives, though men do. Thus, an important part of daily social life for the women centers around the grocery shops. Each grocery has a regular clientele that never goes elsewhere unless an urgent need for an out-of-stock item requires it. Relationships at the grocery are cemented by credit, which usually is extended only to the end of day, and rarely beyond another day or two.

The grocery shops are a socially acceptable setting for women meeting one another, gossiping, exchanging advice, and establishing or extending a social network. The grocery visits are so important that women typically spread their purchases over the morning hours when men are at work, thereby maximizing the time that can be spent with other women at the store without incurring criticism.

Our observations in small groceries over a period of many weeks showed that a wide range of information is exchanged in these conversations: identification of who is a reliable borrower of household items and who is not, opinions on potential marriage partners for children, illnesses and referrals to physicians, means of protection from supernatural or natural risks to mother and child during the first days after a child's birth, and many others. News about events in the homes of near neighbors who are not personally visited comes to women in this way, keeping them well informed about their immediate neighborhood.

The savings group (*gama'iyya*) is a common urban form of informal association, which is not kin-based. While men are increasingly entering into these associations, women are the main organizers and participants. Their commitment to the group overrides any reluctance on the part of their husbands to part with the money which must be contributed periodically. On a rotating basis a designated participant receives the whole fund for some purpose; e.g., key money, furniture or home appliances, marriage or funeral expenses, or schooling. The organizer is a respected woman sought out by the others to form the group, hold the cash, and decide the frequency of rotation, contributions, and who shall be next to receive the fund, all this with consultation among participants. The fund is recreated monthly, or on some other schedule, by everyone making their payment.

The *gama'iyya* not only serves a saving function for members, but is perceived by women as a prior commitment to each other to provide support in time of future need, a need which may or may not be financial. The savings group may be established to last a long time, or only for a short period, and women may be members of more than one concurrently. For many women in the community, participation in such savings groups is an important experience in the movement toward a truly urban form of social relations.

Men's networks

Men also try assiduously to strengthen and widen their networks of social relations. Migrants to the Manshia from Upper Egypt, whether directly or via Cairo, have often obtained their first jobs in the city through kin or regional links, and the same applies for their housing. For example, jobs in the Cairo Bus Authority are particularly accessible to men from Esna in Upper Egypt. Those from Araba in Sohag have extensive links to certain building trades: exterior plastering, house painting, and concrete contracting. Migrants from Fayoum, on the other hand, tend to be unskilled construction workers. These experiences are the initial ones as men build their own networks, many of the elements being employment-based. By marrying one or more sons or daughters to spouses who are from their village of origin, and by placing others in a range of different occupations, both public and private, networks are maintained and expanded.

Today the Manshia resident who needs to borrow money or collect information on how to economize while building a home, who is coping with breach of contract by a business partner, who is considering prospective suitors for his daughter or employment for his sons, or who is simply gossiping to track events, interacts at least as much with co-workers as with neighbors and relatives. His social network is likely to extend far beyond the borders of the Manshia, into many quarters of the city. Place of origin has lost some of its salience though by no means all. By now, the majority of the population of the Manshia is Cairo-born, and patterns of interaction are becoming similar to those of the older urban neighborhoods.

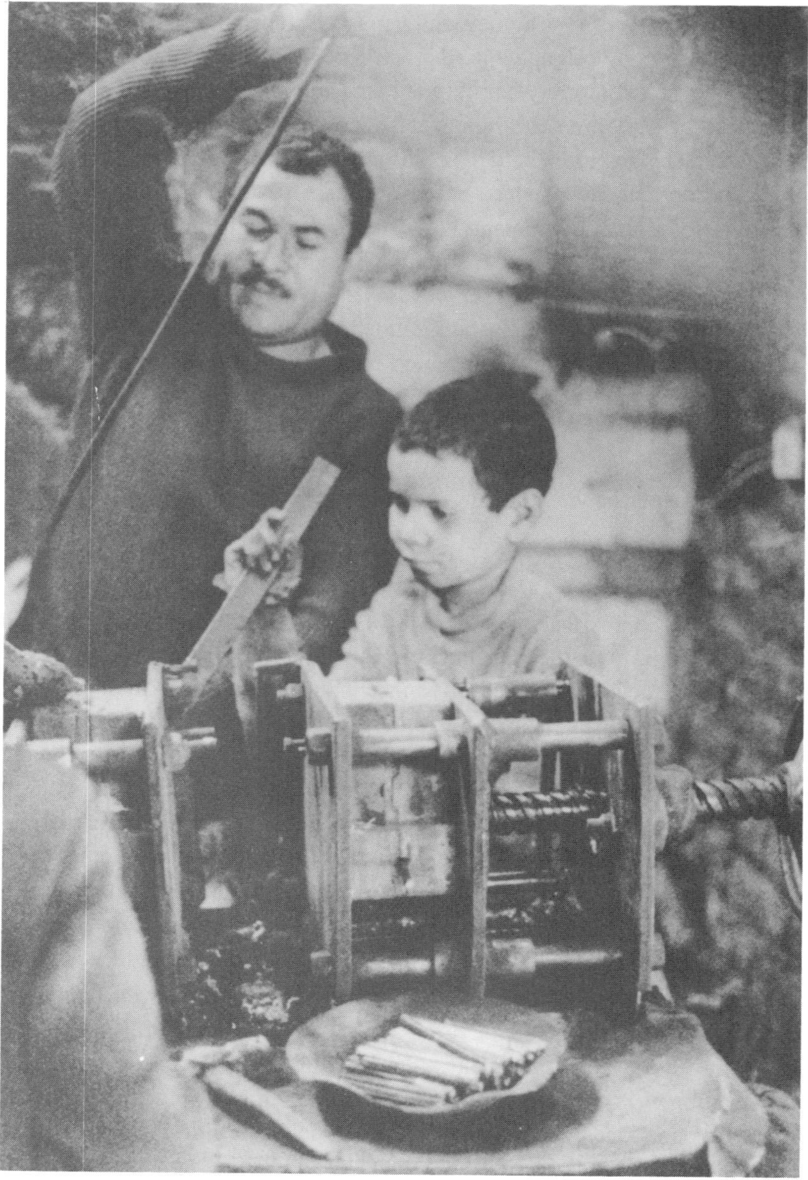

Metal workshop: father and son.

The Arab Council which governed the settlement for many years was itself the epitome of extensive networks. Its most important function was to transform the original settlement from one with very particularistic orientations, and weld it into a community where interaction, in the final analysis, is based on common interests rather than on common origin.

Economic Production in the Settlement

The self-help communities of Cairo are suitable settings for enterprises that can organize themselves to produce efficiently without much relationship to the official state apparatus or the so-called formal sector of the economy. Many such communities have small-scale production and repair workshops, but few show the diversity, vigor, and size that characterizes the small-scale commercial-industrial complex in Manshiet Nasser.

Growing up as a logical extension of the commercial-industrial establishment of the traditional bazaar area in Gamaliya, the Manshia was able to capitalize on the social and economic infrastructure supporting production in the bazaar while being a less expensive area with more space available to the individual workshop. As in the older location, enterprises in Manshiet Nasser tend to specialize in one step in a manufacturing process or trading, then pass the product to others, often nearby, to continue adding value. By the mid-1980s, many industrial and commercial workers who had learned their skills in Manshiet Nasser had spun off to establish their own workshops in nearby communities such as Duweiqa, for exactly the reasons that the proprietors of Manshiet Nasser shops had spun off from those in Gamaliya.

Thus, in keeping with its informality of building and residential arrangements, the Manshia is also part of the ubiquitous informal economy of Cairo. By 'informal' we mean the way in which enterprises conduct their business, having only a limited relationship to laws and institutions that attempt to license and regulate production, set labor standards or organize labor, and collect taxes or fix prices (Castells and Portes, 1989). The activities of these enterprises are not necessarily illegal (although they sometimes are), but are structured to make profits and earn compensation for labor efficiently in an economic environment that offers little appropriate formal support.

The market demand that makes the Manshia's enterprises profitable comes from two sources. First there is the inter-enterprise demand, just discussed, which takes products ultimately to the larger markets of Cairo. Second, a community of this size generates demands of its own for commercial, service, and construction activities to take care of the needs of residents. Where public infrastructure is lacking, small scale private enterprises tend to substitute for the state in providing services in the form of water vending, pit cleaning, garbage collection, and transportation. There is also an abundance of small groceries; in Manshiet Nasser, the average grocery store serves a clientele of about fifty households, functioning as a communication center for the women in particular. Construction is a continuous and integral part of life, so that skilled building tradesmen and shops for construction materials are particularly numerous.

Table 2-7. Resident working population of Manshiet Nasser by sex and location of work, aged ten and above. Percent

Location of work	Males	Females	Both sexes
In settlement	20	48	22
In Cairo	65	49	64
Itinerant	9	2[a]	8
Outside Cairo	4	1[a]	4
Outside Egypt	2	0	2
ALL	100	100	100
Sample N	1359	102	1461

a. The itinerant females are two peddlers; one of whom is a girl of 11 who helps her father. The only female working outside Cairo is a young woman who helps her brother peddling clothes.

Labor and entrepreneurial inputs

The industrial structure of the Manshia goes on growing as workshops expand their businesses and skilled workers branch out on their own. In 1984, the settlement had over two thousand economic establishments ranging from tiny refreshment stands to foundries, some of them with considerable capital investment relative to their small scale. Thus, there was about one economic establishment for every six residential dwelling units. While diminishing land availability is inhibiting construction of new buildings for commercial and industrial use, this area is so well located that building owners find it profitable to build new floors for residential living in order to free lower floors for use as workshops. In this way, the number of manufacturing establishments continues to grow.

The presence of numerous workshops in or close to residential buildings compromises the quality of the living and working environment in the settlement. Their production activities spill out into the alleys, obstructing circulation of people and vehicles and generating noise, smoke, and fumes. While the workshops provide an economic base for some residents, they also burden the community with industrial pollution in a physical setting which already suffers from poor sewerage and other problems.

A substantial share of the labor input comes from outside the settlement. However, the presence of this active and diversified economic base means that residents of the community itself find some of their own employment within the area. Twenty percent of Manshiet Nasser's employed males work regularly within the settlement area (Table 2-7). Considering the ratio of six households to one enterprise, this means that local residents are providing a significant proportion of the labor themselves.

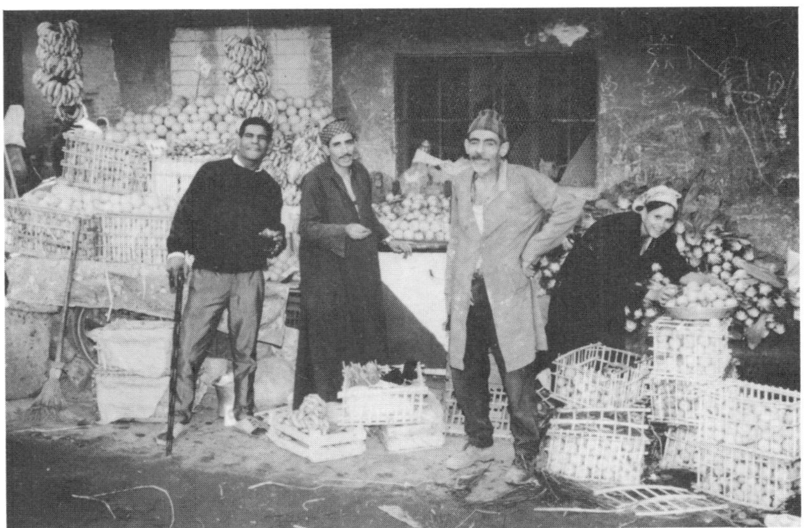

Sellers with a customer. Photograph by Nadir Hashem.

Since the construction trades are an important part of employment for the Manshia's men, one finds many of them at the local hiring halls every day. These are not actually hiring halls in the Western tradition, but coffee shops located near entrances of the community. There, the market is 'made.' Rates and terms are set and men are engaged by employers or clients who need skilled or unskilled workers by the day or for short periods of time. Ragui Assaad (1990a; 1990b) tells us that the men in one such coffee shop function very much like a guild of old, having a structured system of leaders and participation of their 'members'. They are quite successful at accommodating themselves to the realities of wide fluctuations in demand for labor. They have shared norms and practices about apprenticeship, skill classification, and control of entry into the trade that support their own interests.

Some of the enterprises are 'on the street' rather than in buildings as workshops or trading stores. Women work as self-employed or family workers as grocers and greengrocers and as peddlers selling food, bread, drinks, cloth and clothing items, or notions direct to consumers. Most of what they sell is obtained from wholesale sources, but some of their products are home produced, particularly food and some clothing items. The number of such enterprises is not large, but our survey of what women do as part of family support systems, which is reported in the next chapter, showed that 3 to 4 percent of women work in the settlement, many of them in this type of activity.

Workshops of the Manshia that make carpets, clothes pins, shoes, and wires also employ young women as workers. However, except for a limited

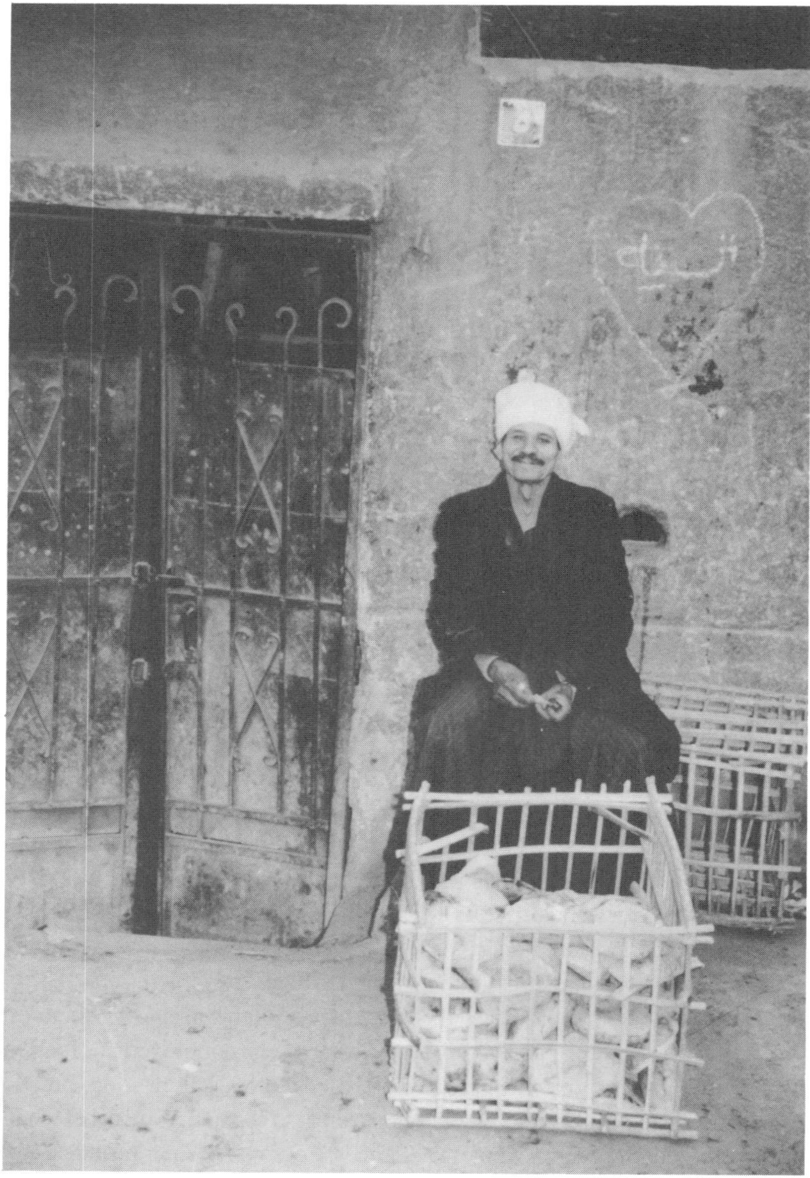

Baladi *bread for sale. Photograph by Nadir Hashem.*

range of enterprises the community's local economy does not offer many opportunities for female labor. Jobs are primarily a male affair within the settlement. Male labor is drawn from outside as well as inside the community.

In some instances, small capitalist enterprises of the settlement use subcontracting to employ women residents for work that they can do at home;

e.g., packaging spices and dried edible seeds, stringing beads, assembling upholstery tacks, painting military medals, and assembling earrings, headbands, and plastic slippers. Women accept this type of work because they do not have the education and skills to compete profitably elsewhere, and because it can be interspersed with regular household tasks and does not separate them from their children. Furthermore, being a home subcontractor involves no expenses for transport or for appropriate clothing to work outside. Since the overall participation of women in cash earning activities, whether at home or in shops, is low in the Manshia, it seems that home-based subcontracting is not a major form of economic production in the community. It is low paid. Women themselves generally negotiate the agreements and determine how the cash income will be used.

Inter-industry relations with metropolitan Cairo

The location of production enterprises, once highly concentrated near the spine road and at the northern end of the settlement, has now spread throughout the settlement area, entering almost every street or alley way. These workshops supply products to the major historic market locations of Cairo, in ʻAtaba and al-Husayn, in the form of brass and alabaster items, gold work, carpets, handmade braiding, spools for thread, shoes, aluminum wares, plastic goods, traditional furniture, and many other items. Some are for final sale by the entrepreneurs who are based both in Manshiet Nasser and elsewhere with an outlet in the city, or are for inter-industry sale, moving along a chain of linked stages of production that add value until the final sale point is reached. Customers are also attracted to Manshiet Nasser from elsewhere in Cairo, for example for car repairs and painting.

A number of the manufacturing establishments also export to Arab countries and the Sudan, using commercial networks strengthened by the contacts of a continuous flow of Egyptian workers and businessmen among the Arab countries. One enterprise was discovered during the study which subcontracts to a Swiss factory. Thus, it is shown once more how the Manshia is by no means a community separate and to itself. Although its inner ways are intensely interesting, it is also part of greater Cairo and the world to which Cairo belongs.

THREE

Manshiet Nasser: Households

Since households are the primary social units within which community and personal resources are gathered, transformed, and used to sustain daily life, it is useful to understand how they are structured and function within Manshiet Nasser. Household organization and composition is governed by widely shared social and cultural norms, but the actual types of households which evolve are quite varied. Their diversity reflects the life stages of different members of the domestic group who are joined together and the resources to which they have access. The subject is, therefore, a relatively large and complex one.

Households are a key layer in the multilayered process of health production. The health and development of young children is immediately dependent on how the household's resources are exploited by its members, especially as they are used by mothers for the bearing and rearing of children. To investigate these matters, three features of households receive special attention in this chapter.

First is the social composition or 'who lives with whom.' This turns out to be a rich subject with a fine texture of variations that can be seen through a combination of quantitative and qualitative approaches. Second are the arrangements for material support of the household. The contributions of men and women are varied dependent upon their role definitions in the setting of the Manshia. We focus selectively on jobs and cash earnings. Third is the human capital that members of the household have acquired through schooling and experience and bring to their activities within the home. Among the members mothers are of special interest because of their central role in the care of children, but fathers also contribute from their personal knowledge and experience, which is taken into consideration as well.

Who Lives with Whom: The Social Composition of Households[1]

Household composition and child welfare

The composition of a household affects its internal functioning through the roles it incorporates within itself. Children and their care is situated within this web of varying complexity. The linkage between composition, which affects how domestic groups function internally, and the health of children

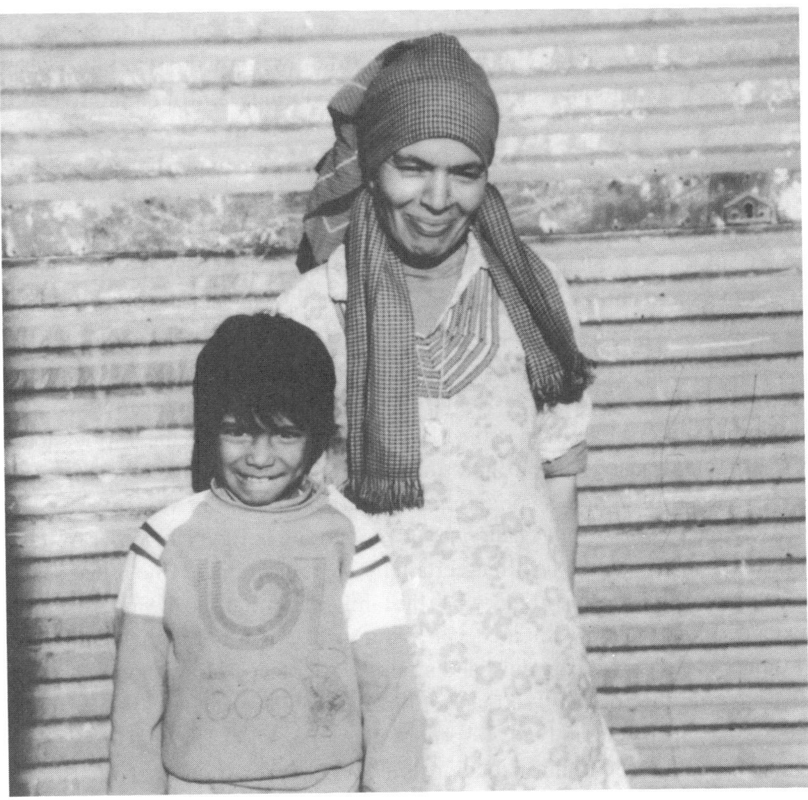

Mother and daughter. Photograph by Nadir Hashem.

has many aspects. The one of particular interest is potential differences in mothering as it is undertaken within different household structures, and the likely affects of these different modalities on child health. It is thought that household structure provides a clue to the position of mothers with respect to management of the household and childcare; and this carries further clues concerning the extent to which there is diffusion or concentration of responsibilities and decision-making power in the conduct of everyday life.

Households also vary in terms of the resources upon which members can draw, who has access, and with what effects on daily lives. The way these resources are used, and thus their health consequences, is affected by the household's membership composition. This is particularly the case for children whose welfare is critically dependent on decisions taken on their behalf by others and especially by their mothers. Personal background and resources of the mother herself, whether they be education, income earning capacities, or neighborhood networking abilities, are all factors that define her ability to command resources on behalf of her children. The presence and the social identities of other persons in the household are also dimensions of competing claims on resources and the intrafamilial power situation. These other persons, including the husband, in-laws, siblings, and other relatives all have their bases of power and claims as well.

A growing body of literature suggests that resources will be assembled and applied more effectively to the production of health for children when their mothers have more rather than less autonomy to perform day to day functions. One problem with this literature is that it draws on the experience of mothers and children in such widely different social settings that general principles do not emerge clearly. Indeed, the content of maternal authority and responsibility, which are both related to autonomy, however it may be defined, has a high degree of cultural specificity. It is useful therefore to examine studies carried out in the Middle East region where the implications of particular household configurations are less divergent, and where we are more likely to find leads concerning what to expect in the Manshia.

One such comes from a national study of fertility in Egypt by Ferial Ahmed (1987: 97–202), where she offers certain incidental findings: One is that death rates among children are higher when the family starts married life in a patrilocal extended household as compared with living on their own. She argues that young women who live with the husband's family are placed in a subordinate and serving role that detracts seriously from their ability to care for their own children.[2] That is certainly one aspect of the story. Another is that extra adult females could offer additional labor time for childcare, for household chores, or provide valuable experience and emotional support when needed. If one sees these large households as systems of dominance and exploitation of the labor power of young wives, rather than as cooperative and supportive groups of people focussed on the welfare of the family and the new generation, then the findings of Ahmed would be consistent. Or there might be other explanations for the findings; they certainly raise an important question.

Cooperation and conflict characterize intrafamilial relationships in simple as well as extended family households; however, there may be particular disadvantages for young wives and mothers under extended family living arrangements. Being more tightly bound within the confines of subordinate role definitions, a predisposition toward stress and conflict is more likely. In an illuminating analysis of the experience and meaning of a folk illness called *'uzr* (spirit possession) in Egypt, Soheir Morsy (1978) hypothesizes that this illness is associated directly with asymmetrical power relations and affords those in subordinate status a legitimate channel for deviating from culturally prescribed behavior patters. She finds that the single largest group of sufferers from *'uzr* are the daughters-in-law living in extended families. For young married women in such households, socially unacceptable behaviors such as neglecting domestic duties, acting contrary to wishes of in-laws, refusing to nurse one's child, and even being childless could only be accepted by claiming and being recognized as *ma'zur* (possessed).

Working in Jordan, Rebecca Doan and Leila Bisharat report that 'in the context of the Arab Middle East, a woman's structural position within the household is a good indicator of her relative autonomy; if she is the daughter-in-law in a vertically extended residential unit, she has less autonomy than if she is head or co-head of household' (1990: 783; also Doan, 1988). Then they confirm statistically that children's nutritional status is worse in such households, relying for their empirical material on data collected from four Palestinian squatter settlements in Amman, Jordan. Controls for income and maternal education were included.

Another study comes from Istanbul, where Akile Gürsoy-Tezcan found higher mortality among children of mothers living in extended families in a large migrant settlement. Her study was based on data from a small survey and in-depth interviewing; information from both sources tended to support her hypothesis. She points out many factors in the dynamics of home environments that she finds are responsible for differential child mortality between extended and simple nuclear households.[3]

Another aspect of household composition in terms of mothering and childcare is the presence of fathers. We are not aware of any studies in this region which have tried to tackle the potentially differential effects on children's health of living in households where there is no father or if he is absent for very long periods. The subject has attracted attention elsewhere, but one must be cautious about transferring hypotheses from one social setting to another.[4] It is also necessary to disentangle income effects on health. To be without a father may imply that the mother loses access to income or other material benefits that the husband could bring, and this could have health effects. It may also precipitate competing time demands on the mother to obtain substitutes for the lost resources. Theorizing should do its best to look at the separate effects of each of these factors on children.

Socialization theory suggests that family functioning is improved when the father is present (McLanahan, 1985). He provides a male role model in relation to cognitive and social development, both of which affect physical development as well, even in very young children. This is the 'father absent' factor in the McLanahan studies and she confirms the negative effects of absence when measuring children's developmental status at school and post-schooling ages in the United States.

For the popular quarters of Cairo, the 'father absent' factor could operate in another rather practical manner. When the father is present, he is often an intermediary in making connections that benefit the family in terms of public goods (including health care) and finding resources or advice needed by the family for various members, including the children. On the other hand, these benefits may be sacrificed over long periods while a father works in one of the oil-rich countries, providing purely material benefits to the family, but not the others.

Belonging to basic family units

As in all human communities, there are rules in the Manshia concerning the composition of households. We shall describe them by drawing a chart which shows the socially permissible moves that individuals may make, or have made for them, from one type of basic family unit to another during the life course. This chart is at the level of the basic units. The way in which they are combined into households is presented later.

The flow of life starts from being a child (see Figure 3-1), born into a basic family unit that is nuclear (whether the household is or not is another matter). The nuclear unit may be broken early by the death or separation of one of the parents, but children always start from a basic family unit that is nuclear. The nuclear units into which children are born are either families headed by their own parents (type **B**) or in some instances broken single-parent units (type **C**) that emerged during pregnancy.[5] From this entry point at the beginning of life, children grow up and make further transitions from one type of basic family unit to another, as shown in the diagram.[6] In this diagram, 'unmarried

Figure 3-1. Life course transitions between basic family units

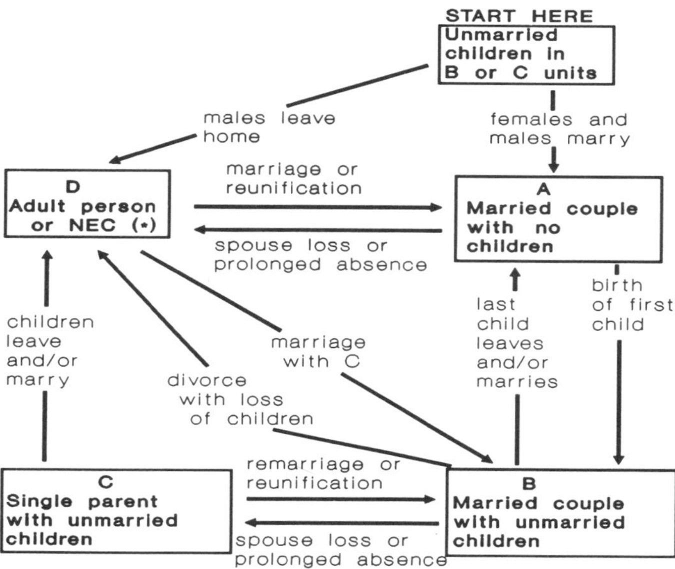

children' means children who are never-married as opposed to ever-married. Ever-married individuals have married at least once, and currently are either married or widowed, divorced, or separated (at some level of recognition by the individuals themselves).

The social rules about who may live with whom operate first of all at the level of basic family units. Secondly, they also govern the grouping of these units into households, or remaining on their own, and these rules are discussed later. The key threshold for a female is to pass from living with parents (or parent) into the married state; this revises her status from being a member of a **B** or **C** unit to being a member of a couple unit (**A**). This change in her basic family status occurs irrespective of whether her household location changes or not. She usually progresses from this state further to having children, which again redefines her status as a member of a basic unit which is couple with children (**B**).

As females grow up the social customs do not allow them to begin their progression by leaving the parental household as unmarried adults. Young males by contrast can do so, but even here, living alone is socially acceptable only if the young man is working or studying at too great a distance for him to be able to live in his parental household. In extreme conditions, such as when both parents have died, a girl or young unmarried woman would at most move to surrogate parents (relatives), and live as a *de facto* adopted child in a type **B** or **C** family unit.

The **D** category is always a single individual; an unmarried male or a divorced, separated or widowed person of either sex whose household does not include his or her unmarried children, although there may be such children living elsewhere. We should mention that the classifications are based on *de facto* living arrangements so that a 'married' woman or man whose spouse is living elsewhere is classified as separated, whether this be temporary or permanent.

Forming households

The principal cultural prescription about household formation is that the socially defined basic family units may be combined in any way, so long as all members of the household are related by blood or marriage. This applies even for young workers living in groups; they should be at least cousins. Some exceptions to this rule are tolerated, but only when strong grounds are present; a few such cases were found in this study. In the Manshia, we did not identify any cases of live-in help, such as might be found occasionally, but not often, in more well-to-do quarters of greater Cairo.

Combinations of basic family units into households are shown by types of households in Table 3-1. The classification proceeds from simple to complex households, and then to the 'no-couple' households that consist of

Table 3-1. Population according to household living arrangements: persons currently living together (*de facto*)

Household compositions	Percent of Total Population	Mean Size of Household
Simple (nuclear) households		
(1) Married couple without children [**A**]	5	2.0
(2) Married couple with unmarried children [**B**]	71	5.2
(3) Single parent with unmarried children [**C**]	6	3.4
Subtotal, simple	81	4.6
Complex households		
(4) One nuclear family (with or without unmarried children) and additional person(s) [Only one **A** or **B** or **C**, with one or more **D**s]	8	5.8
(5) Multiple nuclear families (with or without unmarried children) and with or without additional persons [More than one **A** and/or **B** and/or **C**; with or without **D**s]	7	8.5
Subtotal, complex	15	6.8
No-couple households		
(6) Person residing alone [**D**]	2	1.0
(7) Multiple persons without any nuclear family [two or more **D**s]	2	2.5
Subtotal, no-couple	4	1.5
All	100	4.5
Sample N	4985	1118

one or more individuals among whom there is no pair with a marital tie. The population is distributed among the classifications on a *de facto* basis; membership and thus classification are defined by regular living at home. Persons who are living elsewhere for at least six months, even though expected to return (e.g. migrant workers), are excluded from this description of current household living arrangements. The preference for actual rather than formal descriptions is based on our plan to use this information in discussions of day to day family functioning.

One way to explore the meaning of these classifications is to examine in some detail individual cases chosen more or less at random. The households are selected from the survey records, and a picture is drawn from the information that is contained there. Among simple households, the most typical case is a couple midstream in the family building process:

*Profile of a **B** family living by itself*

The husband, aged thirty-eight, and his wife, aged thirty, have five children. They live in a single-story building which they have built themselves. They occupy one of its two dwelling units, having sold the other one. Their home has three rooms. There is no kitchen as such, and they cook in one of the multi-purpose rooms. The family owns a television set, which is common in the settlement, and also a washing machine, which is a relativley rare convenience, but no refrigerator. They live too far up the slope of the settlement yet to have made a piped water connection. They rely instead on carrying water from other buildings and on the donkey-cart vendor.

They have been married for fourteen years, and moved to the Manshia from the Giza side of Cairo eight years ago. Neither husband nor wife had any schooling, but all of their school-age children are in school. He is said to be receiving an income of LE 272 a month working as a mason in the private-sector construction industry. As long as he continues to get work regularly, they are safely above the median income for lower-income households in the Manshia and Cairo generally.

They started their family with three boys in succession, who are now aged twelve, ten, and nine. Two girls followed, ages six and four. No infants or children have died. Presently, the wife is using the contraceptive pill. This is a basic family unit of type **B**, living by itself as a simple household.

Egyptian family law permits plural marriage for Muslim men. The wives may share a single dwelling or more commonly live separately; our sample shows that 1.2 percent of married women live in households with co-wives, while 5.8 percent of married women had co-wives in other households. The actual rate of plural marriage with separate residence is probably somewhat higher than this, since it is the reports of the wives which are recorded here, and not all wives know when their husbands are also married to another woman. In either event, the man may be establishing long-term, legitimate cohabitation with more than one woman; or he may be replacing the first marriage with a second. In the latter instance, the 'replaced' wife retains the status of a married woman. An example of co-residence of two wives is given next.

*Profile of a type **B** family involving polygamy*

The husband, aged thirty-four, owns a car paint shop. He uses the street as a paint pavilion and has a small room at street level for tools and materials. He has done well and is currently earning LE 390 per month. The household lives in three rooms in a small two-story building which he rents from a relative. The dwelling has piped water.

The first wife, aged thirty, has twin daughters four years old. She has been married fifteen years and has also borne him a son who died later. She is now pregnant with a third child. The husband had a primary education and she had none. Meanwhile the husband has taken a second wife, presently aged twenty-three, who has been educated through secondary school. She has borne two boys in two successive years; the oldest is twenty-one months. His weight for his age is normal, but the two-month old infant is significantly underweight.

No doubt the good income level helps to explain how the man could support a household of this size and complexity. The household is classified as a couple with never-married children (line 2 of Table 3-1). The 'couple' consists of three persons.

The other possibility is that the man has taken the first step in an incremental process that begins with separation and may or may not be followed by divorce. The following illustrates the single-parent household that 'separation without divorce' produces.

*Profile of a type **C** family living in a household of its own*

The mother, aged forty-five, of this single-parent household has a boy of fifteen who works as a baker four days a week. Her daughter of eleven is at home. A third, older child has left home. Altogether, she has been married twenty years and borne eight children, five of whom died. She works herself as a mobile street vendor of peanuts. None of the family went to school.

The woman reports herself as currently married. The husband is a first cousin from her father's side. The husband last visited home two months ago. She says that he has another wife living in a 'parallel' household. She does not consider him to be a member of the household. For her household, the sources of income are her own earnings of LE 52 per month, and those of her son, LE 102 per month.

The household lives in a one-room flat, which it rents. They carry their water from a tap in another building.

When the family (**A**, **B**, or **C**) has an additional relative (**D**) living with it, it is classified as complex (line 4 of Table 3-1). Most commonly, the relative is a mother or mother-in-law, but it can be an aged male parent as well. A woman who loses her husband by separation, divorce, or death may also join the household of a married sibling.

The classic three-generation household may be more interesting and is illustrated next; most of the households on line 5 of Table 3-1 are of this type. The older generation, usually on the husband's side, often prefers that newly married couples start their families with them but other factors work against it. As will be shown below, only about one-third of couples start that way. A major reason is that unless parents own a building that can be enlarged, cramped living space makes such arrangements difficult to achieve.

> *Profile of a three-generation household*
>
> The senior couple of this household consists of a man aged eighty-six and his wife aged fifty-five. They moved from Sohag, in Upper Egypt, four years prior to the study, building their own house in the Manshia. Thus far, the house is a single floor, which they fully occupy. The living situation is relatively comfortable, as the house has four rooms. There is a private toilet with a pit disposal system, but water must be carried from another building which has a tap.
>
> The couple has an unmarried daughter aged twenty-seven and a married son of twenty-two who is a plasterer living with them. Neither offspring received any schooling. The son provides the only visible income of the family, LE 91 per month. Additional unreported resources are likely to exist, as such an income cannot pay for land and construction. Given the son's age and that of his father, it is likely that the family sold land in Sohag in order to buy in the Manshia.
>
> The son married at age eighteen, just before the family's move to the Manshia. His wife was then fifteen and was related to him on his mother's side. She has been pregnant twice, with one successful pregnancy. Their daughter is now twenty months old, but is not in good health, being underweight for her age. The wife is not using contraception, and probably will not do so until she has borne two or three more children.
>
> This household has two basic family units of type **B**, since the older couple also has an unmarried child at home. The household is thus classified as a complex, multi-couple household (line 5 of Table 3-1).
>
> The young couple in a household such as this one is unlikely to split away and establish separate living quarters unless a second unit is constructed in the building where they now live. If the elderly head dies, the household would then become a less complex extended household on line 4.

There are some households in the Manshia without a married couple. These are of two types, those with a solitary person and those with several persons. Since in Egyptian society cultural expectations militate strongly against living alone, there are relatively few of the solitary households that figure so prominently in studies of European populations.[7] When we find people living alone in the Manshia, they are likely to be unmarried young men who have recently migrated for education or work, or married men who need a simple place to live while working, some of them scouting for arrangements to bring their families. If a female is found living alone, she will be an elderly widow in almost every instance, probably in a dwelling inherited or provided by a relative, usually with social support close at hand.

The no-couple households that are formed with more than one person are usually relatively young male workers or students, while others are small groups of older persons who no longer have spouses. In almost every case the co-inhabitants are related to each other, e.g. siblings, cousins, or mother with divorced daughter. Older women usually do not remarry. They constitute a large proportion of the older population classified as type **D**, and some of them live alone or with relatives in households where there is no conjugal couple, i.e. in a no-couple household. One example of a no-couple household is given here. It refers to young persons, exclusively male, living together.

> *Profile of a no-couple household*
>
> Three unmarried brothers from Fayoum aged twenty-two, eighteen, and thirteen live together in a single room rented from the resident-owner of the building. The oldest boy has nearly completed university and will be entitled to a government job after graduation.[8] The next oldest brother completed primary school, dropped out, and is now selling clothing as a full-time street vendor. He does well, making LE 208 a month. The youngest brother, aged thirteen, has not finished primary school. He is currently attending school while also selling clothing on the street. He adds LE 78 a month to the household income.
>
> They manage at minimal expense, cooking on a primus stove and washing up in the courtyard. They have no private toilet or kitchen facility. They carry their water.

These are illustrations of basic family units and their combinations into households that occur in the Manshia. The variety within each type of household is, of course, much greater.

Women's living arrangements during the life course

Another way to look at household composition is from the point of view of the life course of individuals. We have selected to follow the women of Manshiet Nasser and the life-course transitions they experience. To do this, we have developed a procedure that makes use of tables on living arrangements (e.g. Table 3-1) as a starting point. They show the 'average' living arrangements for an amalgam of individuals who are at different stages of the life course (as denoted by their ages). However, someone who is in an extended household at one time may well be in a simple nuclear household at another time or in a single-parent family household at still another stage of the life course. Thus this measure is not, by itself, able to show the likelihood of living in various alternative household formations at different stages of the life course. There are two reasons: the distribution of individuals by type of household is clouded by the particular age and sex composition of the population at that moment; furthermore, the distribution is not even a direct measure of the likelihood of individuals experiencing one of the household formations at a specified stage of their lives. In other words, it lacks the life course perspective.

To achieve a more processual view of the living arrangements of a particular group of individuals (e.g. women) during their lives, we may arrange them by age and the type of household in which they are currently living. Then we form a synthesis of the typical residential situations experienced at each age. The synthesis shows the likelihood of living in a particular type of household as the particular group of persons moves progressively through life. An implicit assumption is that the typical living situation at each age does not change over time, so that all cohorts of women have the same life-course experience. The data fall short of showing all the transitions into and back out of particular states. Nevertheless, the likelihood that women will be found in a particular household formation at various stages of the life course is learned. This likelihood is connected closely to the particularities of the sociocultural definitions of gender and rules of coresidence in the setting of Manshiet Nasser.

The contemporary view of female gender in the Manshia is tied very closely to ideas of motherhood and service to husbands, and also in significant ways to close kin—on both sides. This view is based on a sincere belief in the naturalness of gender constructions. The differences between genders in terms of sentiments and actions are believed to reflect biologically grounded differences between the sexes. Women are defined by their place in the family and their actions are regulated in terms it. This affects the planning and consummation of marriage and living arrangements.

Marriage is an arrangement between families as well as between partners, whether the families are previously related or not. The formation of the conjugal bond does not lead to privatization of family life as it might in some cultures. It entails increased family commitments, and everyone in the relational group is expected to help make the marriage and the new family succeed. In many instances, it also entails strife, with relatives lining up with one partner or the other at times of conflict. Here is a major theme in Egyptian life and literature.[9] For children, being surrounded by relatives is an important environmental fact; it may provide support for their development, but it often generates conflict and ambiguities concerning authority as well.

For women, marriage is the first opportunity to leave home.[10] While it is possible to move before marriage to the home of another relative, if necessity

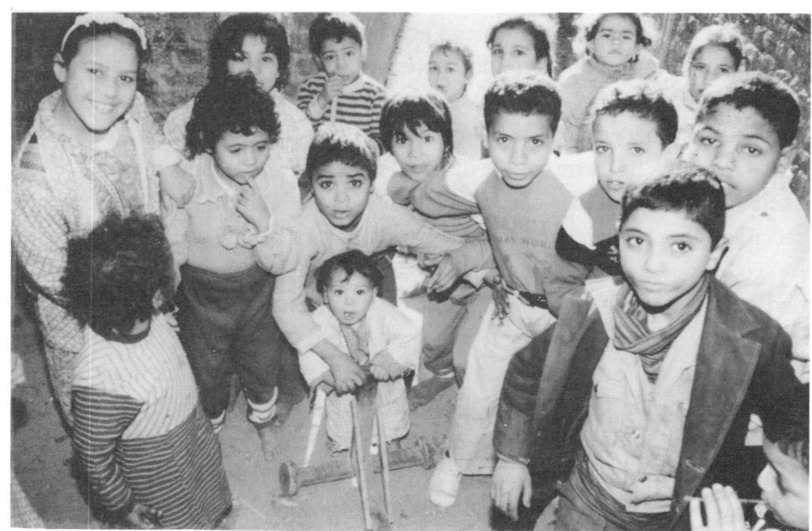

Children of the Manshia. Photograph by Nadir Hashem.

demands, unmarried women are not allowed to live without the protection of kin. Marriage itself usually means a new home, but even that home may be the husband's family household. The husband may also be a relative.

In Cairo as a whole, 32 percent of married women live in consanguineous relationships.[11] There is a class differential; Cairene women without a primary education report themselves to be in consanguineous marriages to the extent of 35 percent. In Manshiet Nasser, marriage to relatives is an even more common experience. Fully 44 percent of married women were married to a relative. Of those related, 70 percent were to first cousins, and in two out of three cases they were paternal cousins.[12]

While there is a substantial body of literature on the functions of endogamy, there is less information about its effects on conjugal relationships, particularly on women's relationships to their husbands and children. Recently within gender studies, the relationship of endogamy to women's position in the family has been gaining analytical importance. Some argue that endogamy reinforces the control of the husband over the wife who has no separate domain of kin relations to rely upon while others argue that it weakens or diffuses this control because mistreatment would alienate one's own kin.[13]

It is also suggested that young women living in extended families are less likely to be harshly exploited or mistreated by their mothers-in-law who are already related to them by other kin ties. Yet it is also possible to argue that these kin ties strengthen the control of the mother-in-law over the young wife, reinforcing her subordinate role and exploitation; leading to double subordination of the young wife in a sense. Consanguineous marriages may also mean less particularization of the mother–child relationship as it becomes embedded in a web of overlapping kin claims. The issue of how endogamy affects conjugal and maternal roles of women is a complex one and the analytical findings to date are ambiguous.

Match making at the time of marriage also conditions the mode of family functioning that will follow, thus influencing management of the household. One of the parameters of husband–wife relationships is the significantly higher age of husbands. On average, husbands are eight years older than their wives in the Manshia. Men's age differences are said by many women to be welcome and to be an advantage for their marriages. However valuable his more mature status in the family network and community, his seniority reinforces (i.e., overlaps with) gender role assignments and hierarchical authority. One implication is the more complete assignment of women to child rearing, without much participation, if any, by husbands.

Living with parents or 'splitting' to live independently

The prospect of marriage raises for every couple the question of where they will reside and start their family. While the cultural context appears to favor living with kin, this may be interpreted as living near to and with the support of kin, particularly when referring to urban environments. In the countryside, 40 percent of all marriages begin with residence in an extended household, generally that of the husband's parents (Ahmed, 1987). Many other newly-married couples, though housed separately, live in close proximity to the parental households. While living with, or in close proximity to parents, is preferred in Cairo too, particularly among the parental generation, it is much less often achieved, and one of the important reasons is constraints on housing.

Preference for the extended family environment is likely to be particularly strong during the first pregnancy and nurturing of the first child. However, several factors work toward an eventual split from complex household living. One is the need for more living space as a new family grows in size. Another is the aspiration of the young wife, and often her husband as well, to manage their own household. The demand for control over home life, its management, and the self-fulfillment that this brings are strong motivations to urge the option of separate residence. A time factor often intervenes so that resources can be accumulated to afford a separate household.

The Cairo data show that only about one-third of young married couples start married life with parents. This includes families of Manshiet Nasser, but by the time they move to the Manshia, they are more likely to have split; indeed, the move itself is often the split. Thus, we find rather low percentages

Table 3-2. **Couples living alone as nuclear families and those living with parents or other relatives by number of children ever born: metropolitan Cairo, 1980. Percent**

Children ever born	Living Alone	With two parents	With one parent	With other relatives	All couples	N
0	64	22	10	4	100	102
1	68	19	6	7	100	176
2	73	10	10	7	100	149
3 +	80	7	6	7	100	156

Note: To investigate 'splitting', we excluded from the universe those couples who were married ten or more years. This avoids contamination of the results by excluding, as far as possible, couples who are living separately because their parents have died thus allowing separate residence to occur without a deliberate split. Also excluded are couples married five years or more who have had no births. They are presumed to be sterile; thus, the number of children (parity) is not genuinely associated with whether the couple lives separately or not.

Source: Data are from the 1980 Egyptian Fertility Survey.

of mothers in the Manshia bringing up children within extended-family households. Nevertheless, the extended family network is crucial to most households in the Manshia. Families make what are often heroic efforts to acquire their own buildings in order to be able to house their sons after marriage, but the majority cannot do so. Dwelling units are typically small, and thus children must be housed elsewhere from the very outset of marriage. Some particularly successful men are able to keep their daughters in the extended household by providing additional rooms for the new couple. Our survey showed a number of such examples in the Manshia.

The justification for splitting grows with the number of children who are born, and as time passes resources may also be accumulated to make the split possible. The process can be seen in Cairo when data on living arrangements are related to the number of children in the family (Table 3-2). The proportion of couples living separately from parents and other relatives rises from 64 percent when there are no children to 80 percent when there are three or more. Much of the savings of migrant workers returning from the Gulf is invested in establishment of a separate household for the nuclear family, in both urban and rural communities, with the Manshia as no exception.

Among those young wives who are still living in complex households, it is common for a mother-in-law or mother to be present; in complex households 30 percent of young wives live with a female parent, either her own or her husband's.[14] Many of these older mothers are not there as support, but to receive support. In some instances, the young couple had set up on its own, but was later joined by the mother.

Table 3-3. Women whose unmarried children are living with them and the proportion of these mothers who are raising their children in nuclear-extended or multiple-couple households, by age of woman. Percent

	By exact age of woman[a]			
Women's living arrangements	**30**	**40**	**50**	**60**
Women whose children are living with them	94	95	84	49
Proportion of these women who are living in complex households	11	12	27	22
Sample N (universe is all women)	379	190	116	57

a. Data for ten-year age groups are centered on exact ages to show percentages against age.

During the middle years of life, almost all women are mothers and live with their unmarried children at home. Until they are forty years of age, about 95 percent are in this state (Table 3-3), after which children begin to leave home one by one. The high prevalence of this type of household arrangement lasting long is due to continued childbearing without early termination, in combination with the social rule that children, particularly girls, do not leave home until marriage. Even as late in life as age sixty, approximately half of women have one or more unmarried children still at home. Girls have generally left earlier by marriage, but boys marry at higher ages, and there is also the not uncommon practice of keeping one son at home for an extended period if he is willing to provide support and protection for the mother.

During mid-life not many mothers who have children at home also have relatives with them; only 12 percent of mothers in the Manshia are in this situation. However, as they pass age forty more and more relatives join them, so that the proportion living with relatives in complex household formations doubles by age fifty (Table 3-3). Even though most women had split from parents and gained independent management of their own households early in married life, reintegration of relatives into some of their households comes along later; either the relatives settle in the couple's home or the couple moves to another relative's home to take advantage of good housing or for some other reason. Partly this is a natural sequence, because women seldom withdraw completely from contacts with the extended kin network, even while pursuing independent management of their separate households. When close family members need to join, or be joined, the predisposition is there.

The proportions of women who become part of complex households rises as their role of taking care of unmarried children diminishes; either children marry but stay in the home for a while, or an offspring who loses a spouse returns, or the older parent generation is by then becoming elderly and joint formations are organized. Among women sixty-five and over, 60 percent have made this transition to complex households.

By this time late in life, the number of women who have survived is declining. In Cairo, only about two-thirds of women successfully survive from marriage to age sixty-five (mortality tables of the 1980s); it is less in Manshiet Nasser. For the survivors, the latter part of the life course often brings widowhood,[15] or it brings separation or divorce when husbands leave their wives for younger women.

There is a dramatic difference in marital experience by gender in the later years of life. At age sixty, a man's probability of being in a married state in Manshiet Nasser is 97 percent, irrespective of his having faced or initiated earlier losses of a spouse. For women it is only 42 percent. Widowhood is high; 51 percent of women by age sixty are widows who have not remarried. When women are widowed, their chances of remarriage are severely limited if they have unmarried children at home or if they have reached age forty to forty-five, which is considered unsuitable for marriage for women.

These marital and demographic developments over the life course mean that many older women have serious problems finding the material and emotional support they need. The subject of women's welfare at older ages deserves study as it is a neglected area in the literature of Egypt. It cannot be assumed, for example, that the system of extended family living, useful as it is, provides well for all or most older women; many family cycles do not play themselves out as in the ideal, and the cities are a particularly difficult place to keep all the linkages among survivors strong.[16] Although women have a normative claim to support and protection by sons, they are aware of its uncertainty and gradual erosion.

The following comments are from younger women speaking about the role of their own children in relation to old-age prospects. They, and sometimes their husbands as well, say that in the old days boys could be counted on, but that now most of them are 'useless.' It is the girls who can be counted on to love their parents, share their lives, and lastly, take care of them when they are old. This perception, even if it may not accord perfectly with reality, is very likely a factor that lies behind our findings much later in this book that girls seem to be brought up as well in terms of health as boys. Different care is given in some respects as we shall see, but with apparently similar results.

Families with only one parent

When children are still growing up, there is a surprising amount of living with one parent, nearly always with the mother. She has lost her spouse for one reason or another, permanently by death, divorce, or separation, or for long periods due to the husband's residence abroad for work. We say surprising, because nuclear family groupings, on their own or within extended households, are usually idealized as if they were the typical, almost universal, environment in which young children are born and reared. The likelihood of single parenting, as we have termed it, is best measured by considering the life course rather than the living arrangements of the whole population at a particular date in time. Nevertheless, as a starting point, before moving to the life-course point of view, it may be noted that the population living in single-parent families on their own is 6 percent of the population of all ages and both genders (Table 3-1). To this should be added those people who are living as single-parent family groups within complex households. In the Manshia, for every five one-parent families living independently, two more are living within complex households. The social connotations and consequences of these two types of living arrangements are likely to be quite different.

For a significant proportion of mothers, long absences of husbands for work during their child-rearing years place them in *de facto* single parenting situations. We have assigned this status only for absences of six months or more, treating short absences as current residence.[17] The meaning for them of such single parenting is different from permanent dissolutions, but the day to day context is not so greatly different for the children.

The ideology of kin relations and views about proper female behavior would suggest that mother–child family groups should be absorbed into other larger households where they could be under the protection and support of adult males. If the mother is relatively young, she does not usually live separately unless she has at least two children to constitute a socially recognized family. When single parenting is due to extended work abroad by the husband, the decision about where she will live during his absence is largely decided by whether the independent household is already well established as a family; if not, the woman usually moves back to her natal home or is taken into some branch of the husband's family. The wife is likely to oppose her husband's labor migration until her own independent household is securely established. After that point, she may encourage migration for work in order to increase the household's assets.[18]

No simple explanation for finding that the majority of single parent families live alone can be offered, but one observation is worth noting. There is a question of material support. Single-parent families seldom live separately unless at least one member, an older child or the parent herself, is gainfully employed; occasionally there are two earners. Remittances from an absent husband or relative are another possibility. Thus, to continue life in an independent household may be considered preferable, but it must also be affordable.

There are, of course, both females and males who are single parents living with one or more of their unmarried children. The ratio of female to male parents is high: 10 to 1. Given the gender role definitions prevalent in Egyptian society, the one-parent family groups headed by a male do not survive for long. The male remarries or the children are placed with someone else to live. We do not pursue the study of male one-parent families further.[19]

To gain a better appreciation of the likelihood of having single-parenting experiences, one must scan the life course of individuals. From the individual's point of view, this is the relevant information, i.e. the prospects of being a single parent whether one is at the moment or not. From an individual woman's point of view, the probability of becoming a single parent exists only after marrying and beginning to bear children. This probability rises with the duration of the marriage. Separation from the spouse and final dissolution occurs with the playing out of the marriage history, unless the husband predeceases her or all the children grow up and are married first. A mother may enter the state of being a single parent, leave that state when reunited with her husband or remarried, and leave it finally with the marriage of all the children.

Because the progression of residential states is not unidirectional, without return to a former state, information on the current state of women at different ages does not tell us about the cumulative number of women who have had the experience. As age rises, the information misses more and more women who have had the experience but are no longer in that state. Indeed at very high ages, no women are in a single parent state and yet many of them have had the experience. Nevertheless, we may look at the proportions of women in a single-parent state as age increases (Figure 3-2).

Figure 3-2. Women's probability of being lone parents with unmarried children at home by age of woman

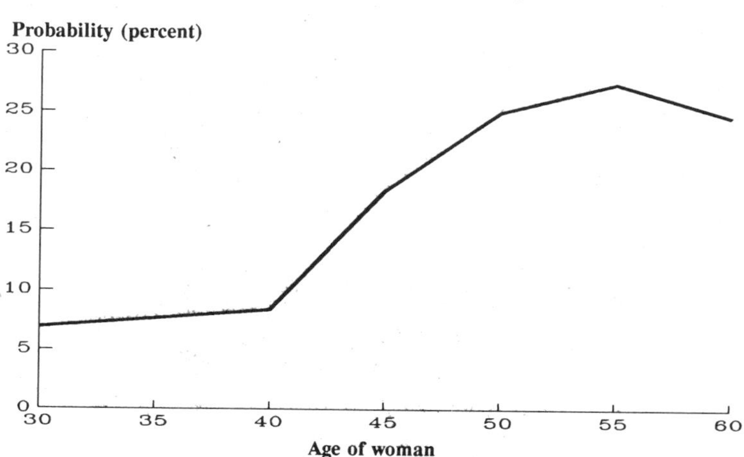

Note: Women at risk are all women who have ever married.

Table 3-4. Distribution of children (never married) between simple and complex households by age of child. Percent

Age group	Simple	Complex	Children N
0-4	89	11	1083
5-9	87	13	783
10-14	80	20	472

Note: Simple and complex households are defined in Table 3-1.

The probability curve rises by age as partners are lost for one reason or another and not replaced or reunited. The probability is remarkably high at the older ages when one would expect the phenomenon of the 'empty nest' to occur, and single parenting to cease. These older women are mostly mothers who still have at home late-marrying children supporting them. The number is small, however, because practically all men and women eventually marry in Egypt. As fertility declines in urban communities, the last-born will be born at younger and younger ages of mothers, so this older-age type of single-parent family is likely to diminish.

The highest point on the probability curve (27 percent) is an under-estimate of the proportion of women who have ever experienced single parenting, because the statistics are not cumulative. Some of these women have entered the single-parent state earlier in life and then exited that state by re-marrying, reuniting, or seeing all their unmarried children marry and/or leave home. The actual probability of ever being a single parent, therefore, is higher. How much higher has not been measured.[20]

Children's living arrangements

In a study concerned with child health, it is interesting to examine, from the child's point of view, where they live during their early years. The story of where children live during their early years is constructed by examining how children are distributed among households of different types, keeping the ages of the children in mind. The broad division between simple and complex households is used in Table 3-4, submerging for the moment any reference to living with one parent. The environment of the simple household predominates overwhelmingly; very few of the children are being reared in complex households it would appear. Because some of the children began their lives elsewhere in Cairo, before the parents moved to the Manshia, some information on living in complex households has been screened out. Nevertheless, one is impressed by the dominance of the simple nuclear-family form of living arrangement for young children.

Figure 3-3. Children's probability of living in a single-parent family by age of the child

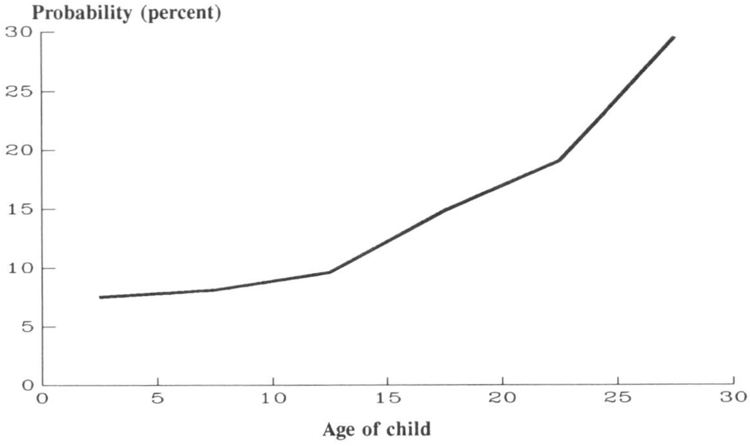

Probability (percent)

Age of child

Note: Children at risk are children who have never married.

The downward drift of the proportion of children living in simple households as they get older is mainly due to the progress of the life cycle of parents. The first-born generally escape the transition, and leave home by marriage or, if boys, also for work or education. The last-born are in the household as it matures fully and becomes a potential place for grandparents or aunts to live if they have lost their own partners, or for some other reason.

From the children's point of view the probability of having only one parent at home is almost negligible at birth. It rises as they get older in association with the mother's risk of single parenting which rises with her passage through the life course. Last-born children are more likely to experience life with only one parent simply because the parents' marriage is at a later stage. The curve showing the probability of children being in a single-parent living environment rises with age as shown in Figure 3-3. In this figure, the number of children subject to the probability declines with age as they marry and/or leave home.

For boys and girls there is no difference in risk up to age fifteen or so. After that, as girls leave home for marriage while boys marry at older ages, a differential risk develops. By the early twenties, boys outnumber girls two to one. Living with a lone parent means different things to boys and girls. Often the boys are involved in providing income support to the single-parent family. Indeed, their presence with its image of male protection, is sometimes a factor permitting separate living for single-parent women.

How Households Support Themselves

Another aspect of the household that affects its functioning and capacity to achieve health for its children is the means by which material resources are obtained. As in most societies, there is clear gender-specific role differentiation in the Manshia. It is primarily men who work for cash outside the home, as employees, self-employed laborers, and small businessmen. Women also work in family business and even elsewhere, but in much smaller numbers. Their main economic contributions are the creation of material goods or services for the household through housework and home production. A central defining trait of the ideal wife and mother, for example, is her ability to conserve resources by restricting expenditures.

Since many basic commodities are supplied through special outlets at subsidies as part of the government's policies for keeping a floor under the poor, women are usually the family member responsible for queuing and making timely visits to the supply points. Men may help by bringing goods from their workplaces. Health care and education are in principle available at no more than token costs from government or private voluntary organizations, but there are costs in time and for supplementary items to make the services useful. Thus, the appropriation of public goods may be advantageous, but it is not free of cost. Bringing material goods and services into the household includes this appropriation activity. Similarly, but in an entirely different domain of relationships, receiving assistance from relatives and close friends, as well as giving assistance is also part of the process. Women are primarily responsible for both, though certain transactions fall to men as well.

Working for cash: men and women

The principal breadwinner of a household may be defined as the member who earns more than any other member, usually more than one-half of the household's cash income. This person is typically a male who is almost invariably reported as head of the household; the only exception would be an elderly father no longer working but still recognized by the family as its head. However, there are enough exceptions to this 'ideal type' to warrant attention. For example, in 9.4 percent of households in the Manshia, a woman is the principal breadwinner, even if not the official head of the household in most instances. Or if not the principal breadwinner, she may be a contributing earner of cash. Furthermore, children often work for cash in workshops, on the street as peddlers, or in family businesses.

To convey an idea of what kinds of work are done by people of the Manshia, a list of jobs was compiled by taking a systematic representative sample from all the jobs that were found in the survey. Certain jobs repeat themselves in the list, because every job holder had an equal chance of selection (Table 3-5). There are

Table 3-5. Profile of labor force: representative sample of job descriptions by age, sex, and earnings

Job description	Age	Sex	Monthly earnings LE
Aluminum metal works, owner	34	Male	315
Baker	28	Male	156
Bread salesperson	35	Male	60
Car paint shop, owner	34	Male	390
Carpet factory worker	14	Male	52
Clothing vendor (mobile)	22	Male	182
Contractor	36	Male	481
Draftee	19	Male	6
Electrician	26	Male	234
Laborer, construction	35	Male	250
Laborer, construction	40	Male	143
Laborer, construction	35	Male	94
Laborer, construction	29	Male	102
Laborer, construction	52	Male	70
Gold salesperson	14	Male	130
Guard	42	Male	100
Janitor	32	Female	50
Mechanic weaver	42	Male	130
Notions salesperson	60	Female	200
Painter	18	Male	105
Plasterer	35	Male	234
Policeman	34	Male	65
Railway conductor	35	Male	120
Seamstress	23	Female	31
Sweeper	40	Male	60
Tile layer	22	Male	182
Turning lathe operator	38	Male	130
Upholsterer	49	Male	136
Workshop (unspecified), owner	27	Male	260

Note: At the time of the survey, the Egyptian Pound had a foreign exchange value of approximately one US dollar. The data are a 1-in-50 representative sub-sample from the main survey sample.

owners of workshops as well as employees and self-employed workers. The differences in monthly earnings illustrate the point that participation in the informal economy does not equate with poverty. It also shows the high variation of earnings in the informal sector. Indeed, to be a policeman or railway conductor, connected with a large and formal organization, does not seem to be an outstanding advantage in terms of carry-home cash.

Work for cash begins early in life, particularly for boys. Nearly 30 percent are working below age fifteen (grouped data for 10–14 in Figure 3-4). One of the reasons is the general failure of technical trade schools to attract young persons, because they do not lead to jobs. Boys are more successful when they apprentice at an early age to workshops, factories, or to the construction trade either in Manshiet Nasser or in nearby districts. The rest of Figure 3-4 is more or less what one expects to see in urban communities settled by people with first or second-generation migrant backgrounds and low educational qualifications. Women have few options for cash work that genuinely pay more in cash (after expenses) than they can save for the family by home production and management. In addition, there is family rearing which does not mix well with outside work. The somewhat elevated female employment rates at the higher ages is due to women's loss of access to male wages when widowed or separated and, therefore, fewer duties at home.

It is well accepted by the community that girls with education to the secondary level be employed, and it is also acceptable that women who are heads of households, such as the older women, be employed or generate income. People are still quite concerned about uneducated girls, or married women, being employed, and prefer that it not occur except in family business. In the Manshia, women who are working say so, rather than try to hide it. This seems to be distinctive, because one finds less disclosure in some of the other communities, out of shame for the anomaly in their behavior.

Where people work is also of interest. Women are much more likely to arrange for work near at hand in the community, because this combines well with their other activities. It avoids the additional costs of transportation and special clothing suitable to the more urbane environment elsewhere in the city. Furthermore, the tasks they would have to pass to others or leave undone, including childcare, are a negative factor in the balance of their choosing not to work. Furthermore, if she does journey outside the settlement, the workplace must be a place where no rumor or speculation about her character or her collegial relations will arise.

The employment opportunity structure offers the Manshia's women very little elsewhere in the city, given their own qualifications and the bias against

Figure 3-4. Gainfully employed residents of Manshiet Nasser by age and sex

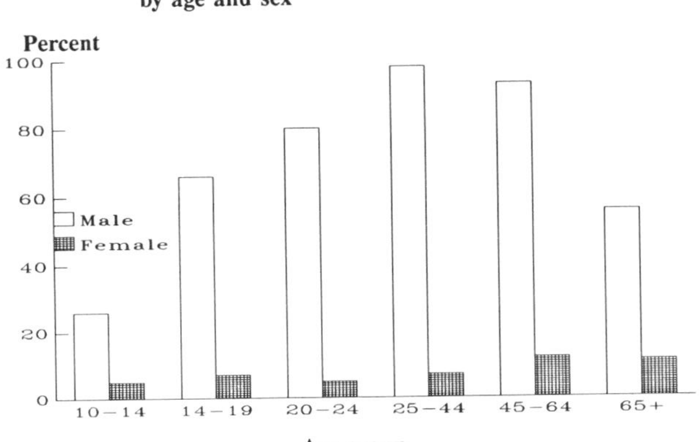

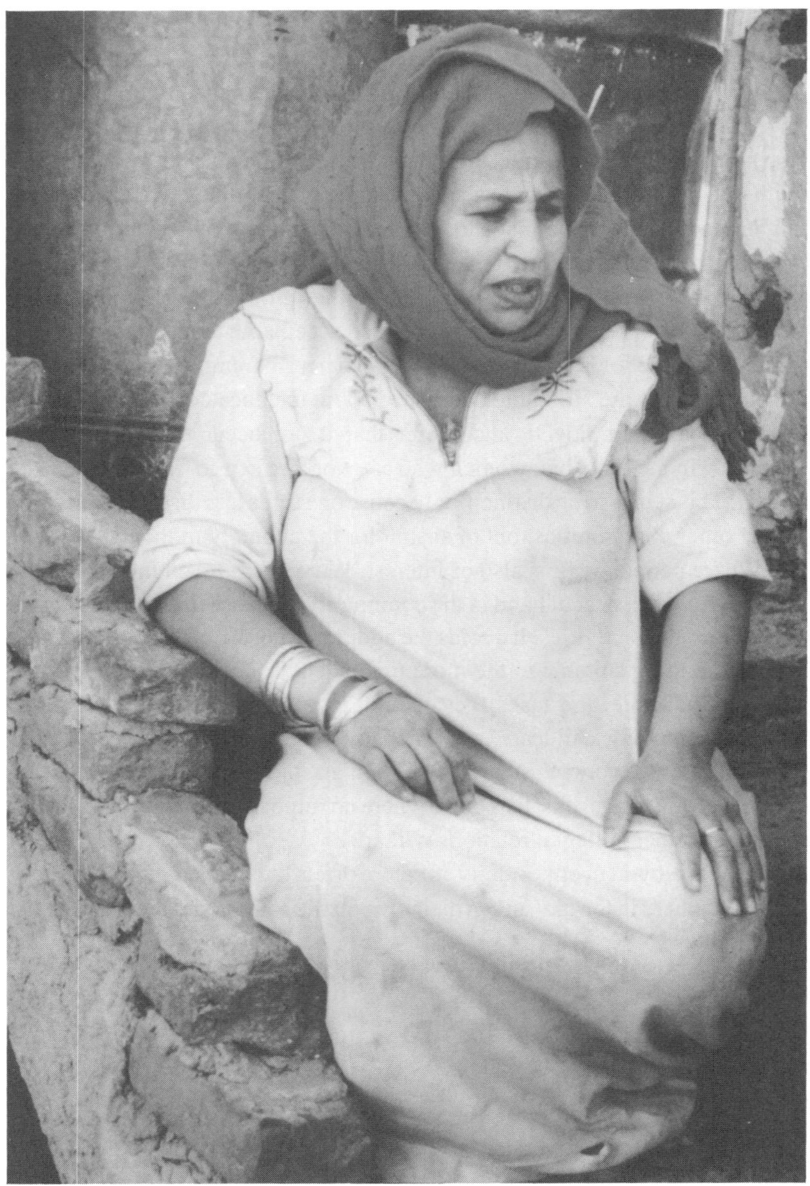

Grocer. Photograph by Nadir Hashem.

female employment in many types of work. Men, on the other hand, go where the best jobs are to be found, because they are expected to be the breadwinners and are not constrained by tasks at home. Only 20 percent of the male labor force works within the Manshia (see discussion in previous chapter of the economic organization of Manshiet Nasser, particularly Table 2-7).

When women work in family businesses, as they sometimes do with their husbands, it should not be seen solely as exploitation of cheap family labor. In some of these jobs, such as food preparation and vending, or greengrocer retailing, women's capabilities come forward and the interaction with husbands produces a more egalitarian relationship in other areas of family functioning as well.[21]

The community is both too new and has too few residents with the minimum educational qualifications to be strongly tied to public-sector employment. In the Egypt of Gamal 'Abd al-Nasser, such employment was an important goal, because that is how the economy and future security for individuals were organized. With the advent of new policies, particularly the 'open door' to international transactions and its privatization tendencies, the employment structure and its rewards have changed. There has been a general deterioration in public-sector remuneration as compared with private earning levels.[22] Private employment, including self-employment, has become preferable in terms of current income and flexibility of options.

Nevertheless, government employment, although poorly remunerated by comparison with private (which is confirmed by our income data for Manshiet Nasser), still offers types of health, old age, and disability benefits that people value. For women it is an option that offers a respectable job and some security against adversity should she lose her husband later in life. For men, whose family roles do not keep them at home, government work is often combined with overtime or second-job activities. While some women are thus working in the bureaucracy, they are rarely found in production or service jobs of the public-sector enterprises.

When the job arrangements are inspected (Table 3-6), there is not a great deal of difference between men and women so far as the public–private dichotomy is concerned. However, within the private sector, women are noticeably more engaged in self and family employment than in working for

Table 3-6. Working population of Manshiet Nasser by sector of gainful employment and sex, aged 10 and over. Percent

Sector and employer	Males	Females
Private		
Self, family	25	48
Other private	54	35
Public		
Government	15	15
Public enterprises	6	2
All employed persons	100	100
Sample N	1378	104

non-family persons. This may be linked to the view that working in family enterprises or as 'market women' selling food, drinks, groceries, and notions on the street is a natural extension of their female aptitudes and responsibilities, and therefore easily accepted socially. The prevalence of such jobs is also due to the opportunity structure for women, which offers them few other options.

Household income

It is notoriously difficult to obtain good estimates of cash income from surveys. To minimize this problem, the survey did not ask directly about the income levels of the households. Rather, it collected data on jobs, days worked, and places of work. Estimates of the cash incomes that go with specific jobs were then collected from independent informants in the community, including workers in the trades in question and employers. The rates were cross-checked by interviews in similar communities elsewhere in the city. For persons who are self employed or in family businesses, an element of profit or return on business capital was included in our estimates of cash earnings.

This approach produces a higher but arguably more realistic estimate of incomes than can be achieved through direct questioning. It should be kept in mind, however, that this method of assessment is different from that used in other surveys of income in Egypt and makes the Manshia appear somewhat more affluent relative to statistics for Cairo as a whole than is really the case.

For 10 percent of households there was no gainfully employed person, so earned income was recorded as none. Either these households were living on property incomes or on transfers from their own savings or relatives. Employable members of the family could have been between jobs, but currently without income. Or we simply had a case of failure to obtain an accurate report from the respondent. The profile of income which is presented in Table 3-7 excludes these cases of no visible earned income. The result may be an upward-biased picture of income, but this is preferable to presenting one which would be downward-biased by inclusion of the doubtful cases.

Table 3-7. Profile of the household income distribution: monthly incomes in 1984

Households ranked from highest to lowest income (Percent of households)	Percent of all income	Range of incomes LE	Median earned income LE
Top 20 percent	35.3	234 +	260
Next 20	28.9	143-234	182
Next 20	15.0	104-143	130
Next 20	12.9	75-104	90
Bottom 20 percent	7.9	Up to 75	60
ALL (N = 1007)	100.		130

Note: This excludes 111 households for which no jobs were reported.

Table 3-8. Monthly income by household composition: means and standard deviations

Household compositions	Number of house-holds	LE per household Mean (SD)	LE per consumer unit Mean (SD)
Simple (nuclear) households			
Married couple without children	117	154 (103)	77 (52)
Married couple with unmarried children	678	176 (121)	53 (34)
Single parent with unmarried children	85	142 (119)	55 (40)
Single parent is female	*76*	*140 (123)*	*52 (39)*
Complex households			
One nuclear family (with or without unmarried children) and additional person(s)	69	216 (173)	52 (38)
Multiple nuclear families (with or without unmarried children) and with or without additional persons	41	291 (201)	44 (26)
No-couple households			
Person residing alone	88	77 (72)	77 (72)
Multiple persons without any nuclear family	40	216 (234)	87 (77)
All	1118	171 (135)	58 (44)

Note: Income is defined as the income of regular residents of the household plus estimated remittances from members currently residing elsewhere. Consumer units are the number of adults plus children (under 15 years of age) weighted as .35 units. All households are included, some of which had no visible reported income.

The level of incomes prevailing in this settlement may be considered against information concerning urban income levels in Egypt as a whole. The comparison shows the vulnerability of the Manshia's households in relation to other urban households. One study (the only one available but a satisfactory one) estimates the average monthly household income at the poverty line for urban Egypt to be LE 183 per month (Korayem, 1987).[23] For Manshiet Nasser the median earned household income in the same year (1984) is LE 130. Evaluating the extent of vulnerability by looking at the proportion of households falling below the poverty line, this proportion is 64 percent for Manshiet Nasser.[24] Evidently, the Manshia is a community that straddles the poverty line, but has more households below than above it.

One should take care not to assess the income levels of households as if all were similar, when there are substantial differences in size and in the types of individuals grouped within them. A more finely drawn picture is presented in Table 3-8. Size is taken into account by spreading earned income over consumer units, defining adults as equal to one unit and unmarried children under age fifteen as .35 units. While the assignment of weights in this fashion is arbitrary, the choice of weights rests on the observation that the Egyptian subsidy system for basic consumer items and for health care holds down the cost of rearing children as compared with expenditures for adults. Education costs have begun to climb with the employment of tutors in the Manshia, but so far fees are low.[25] Studies in countries where child-rearing costs are higher generally use higher coefficients.

The complex households have significantly larger income flows than simple households. Among the no-couple households, which are a third category, those with multiple persons do well (last line of table). They are mainly groups of male workers. Their average size is smaller (2.5) than that of the complex households (6.8), but work is their reason for existence and, not surprisingly, they earn as much as many of the larger complex households.[26]

When income is calculated on the basis of consumer units, the difference between complex and simple households essentially disappears. There are two exceptions. Couples who do not yet have children (first line) are temporarily ahead, but that differential soon disappears in the course of the life cycle. At the other end of the life cycle for many people are those two-couple, usually three-generation, households designated as multiple nuclear families. They carry a disproportionate number of adults who no longer have visible earned incomes. It is typical of household income statistics that they miss the savings, property incomes, and transfers from relatives that often augment the cash flow of such households.

To obtain an idea of trends of income, it is useful to recall that many of the Manshia's workers are directly dependent on the construction trades or their supporting production sectors for work. Thus, earnings trends in this sector are a reasonably good indicator of earnings in the community as a whole. Wage markets in other sectors are not, of course, independent, but are influenced by labor substitution between them and construction. Ragui Assaad's research on the construction labor markets in Egypt is a mine of information about wages and earnings (1989; 1991). He shows how real wages rose by about 60 percent during the first 6 years that followed the boom in labor migration to the Gulf countries, financed by the 1973 jump in oil prices. At home in Cairo, the atmosphere among those who stayed behind, as well as those who migrated for work, was optimistic because of the buoyant labor markets, and the rapid escalation in purchasing power in the general population. Rapid development of the Manshia was a derivative.

The upward trend of real wages faltered at the beginning of the 1980s and wages were declining slowly by the time of our survey. However, in construction, continuous unemployment or frequent days without work had not yet hit the Manshia. Initially, the decline was masked from the population by price inflation for consumer goods and services, because inflation was a relatively new phenomenon not taken into most people's thinking. By 1987, however, about three-fourths of the original gain in real wages had been lost, partly due to Iraq's expulsion of Egyptian workers, so the depression suddenly became much more visible. In 1990 and 1991, massive returns of workers from the Gulf countries caused a general depression in all types of employment except for those in more stable sectors such as government employment, who are not numerous in the Manshia. By then, inflation during past years had thoroughly robbed fixed income recipients of many of the advantages of their secure jobs.

While employment has diversified in the Manshia, which helps to spread risks of interruption of the community's income, it has continued to be insecure and unstable at an individual level. Apart from the real effects on family welfare, which are themselves of concern, there is a statistical implication for the present study. In our statistical modelling below we use measurements of current income differentials at the household level as an independent variable. Irregular income carries the implication that differentials in long-term income are not well measured by current income, even though this may be the best that can be done to approximate an income variable.

The Human Resources of Households

Members of the household provide the labor time, knowledge, skills, and commitment to transform material resources into the health inputs of daily life. All members may contribute to these transformations, albeit in different ways and with different degrees of responsibility for activities that contribute to health. In this section, we are concerned with the processes that produce or enhance the capacities of individual household members, particularly mothers and fathers, to contribute. Among these capacity-building processes are schooling experience and work experience. Though we shall focus particularly on these two processes, we readily acknowledge that parents build their capacities in other ways as well. Socialization in their own families, and work experience are particularly important when the adults have had little opportunity for schooling.

Mothers' education and managerial capacities

Maternal education has been found to be consistently associated with reproductive behavior and child survival experiences of women in a wide variety of social settings. The relationship between women's education and reduced fertility and child mortality remains significant after allowing for other social and economic characteristics of educated mothers (Behm, 1979; Cochrane, 1980; Caldwell and McDonald, 1981; Tekçe and Shorter, 1984; Cleland and Van Ginneken, 1989). The specific mechanisms through which maternal education affects child survival, and the level of schooling at which these relationships become important, are not well understood and evidently vary by cultural context.

The ways in which education of women enables them to manage their homes to the benefit of the health of their children needs to be viewed from a wide angle. We argue that the benefits are not limited to the content of the instruction and information that formal schooling may convey.

First of all, it is important to go beyond the use of mother's education as a simple proxy variable for living standards of the family; in the present study the information on material income of the household (see above) is intended to handle that relationship more directly. Explanations of the role of education in its own right have usually pointed to the skills and knowledge of a more educated woman concerning prevention and treatment of disease. Also, there are status enhancement effects: the family and community usually accord her more authority and independence of action, which enables her to act more effectively on her knowledge. Our argument accepts these points as far as they go, but adds the following: women who have had the experience of schooling tend to develop different definitions of self and their own relationship to others and to the world around them. This enables them to take more deliberate and effective command over existing household resources and their transformation into various uses, many of which are effectively health inputs for their children.

Formal education for females, if sustained until and beyond a socially recognized minimum threshold such as primary schooling is passed, is thought to produce a change in definition of self, and related to this a modified attitude toward one's personal relationship to the environment. This stems from basically two sources. One is that only a special kind of family is likely to encourage a girl to go through several years of schooling in communities where there is reluctance to educate girls and consequently low levels of schooling. One may not be able to identify precisely what the constituent elements of this 'specialness' are, but at a minimum it involves placing a value on developing the capacity of a female child rather than simply viewing her femaleness as a naturally adequate resource for the performance of the only two important roles she is ever likely to play: wife and mother.

Such a family may be relatively better off and be headed by parents who are themselves educated. The substantial contribution young girls make in carrying out the many labor-intensive household chores that need to be done in poor settings, both for the immediate family and for wider kin, competes against schooling. However, her labor time may be fitted around schooling activities, or other family members help out.

We may pause to illustrate. An example of the difficulties encountered in educating female children was seen during the in-depth study of the family of a female grocer in the settlement. Her oldest daughter, aged ten, helps her grandmother who is also a grocer and lives in a nearby settlement. The grandmother is diabetic and the granddaughter spends all the summer and many winter nights with her. When the grandmother was hospitalized for several months during the last school year, it was the granddaughter who stayed with her in the hospital. She barely managed to pass her grade. Since then she has been staying with her grandmother periodically, for weeks at a time, helping out with household chores.

There are differences of opinion among the adults in the family concerning education. The grandmother, that is mother's mother, is of the opinion that education 'dirties the minds of girls' and has always put pressure for her granddaughter to leave school. The mother and father do not make gender distinctions in education but still differ in their approach. The father believes that all children should stay in school and be encouraged to go as far as possible, while the mother thinks that only some children are suited and should be encouraged. It is becoming gradually accepted in the family that some time soon the daughter will go to live with her grandmother to help her and stop going to school altogether. A second, younger, daughter, however, attends school regularly.

Whatever may be the nature of factors that allow school attendance to take place, the ultimate meaning of that experience is that the female child learns to participate in a formal institution of her society outside the nexus of family relationships. This point brings in the second aspect of schooling which is arguably more important than the selectivity of the family of origin. It is proposed here that the experience of formal schooling is the key factor in transforming self images whereby one tends to view the world more as an actor than a spectator. If the premise is accepted that the meaning of the experience is more important than its curricular content, then it is not surprising that whatever may be the physical condition of schools and however deficient the quality of curriculum, formal schooling powerfully differentiates female behavior, including childbearing and childrearing, in a wide variety of settings.

From a sociological perspective, schooling is a learning experience in a much broader sense than in terms of exposure to a formal curriculum. The children also acquire social skills, such as functioning in a group other than that of family and kin, and observe codes and practices governing behavior when interacting with others, such as teachers and fellow students, in distinct non-familial roles. One learns what strategies are acceptable in a classroom, how to respond to those in positions of authority, and acquires a sense of scheduling and periodicity of events. Even the daily trip to school, which most mother's are too busy to chaperon themselves, involves exposures to settings both inside and outside the settlement, keeping in mind that many of the children walk long distances to schools.

The aspect relevant to the behavior of an adult woman is the development of a capacity to organize and influence domestic and external environments, and to seek out new knowledge when needed, in order to achieve desired ends, rather than what she may have learned and retained from school about disease transmission, hygiene, or even literacy. The schooling experience is so powerful because it is not confined to the acquisition of specific knowledge, but increases capacity to take effective action in a multiplicity of situations. It also contributes to structuring of domestic relations such that exchanges with male members are less likely to be sharply unequal.

The development of a more deliberate and active style of mothering seems to require openness to new ideas, a heightened sense of responsiveness to children's needs, and a more interventionist approach to fulfilling those needs, but not necessarily achieving better child health outcomes. The outcome also depends upon what is available to mothers to work with in a specific setting in terms of food, clothing, shelter, sanitation, and health services.

These arguments are consistent with Caldwell's (1979) proposition that participation in formal education changes one's own perceptions of self, as well as the perceptions that others have of the woman. In a similar vein, Ware (1984) notes that only a special kind of family is likely to encourage a girl to be schooled in social settings where this is not the norm; hence, the girl herself becomes strong vis-à-vis the environment around her. For the older women

Figure 5-3. Weights of children by percentile of the normalized NCHS standard Five-month moving average

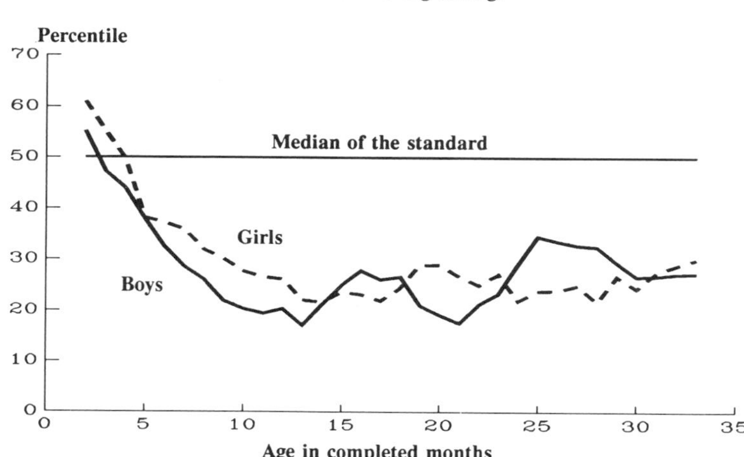

of Manshiet Nasser this rings true. For the new generation there is far less selectivity; the ambition of young mothers is for daughters to complete at least primary schooling.

One can see in the data on women's education (Figure 3-5) that President Gamal 'Abd al-Nasser's educational reforms of the 1950s, including insistence on making education more widely available with reduced gender discrimination, has had an effect. Cohorts that entered primary school in the 1960s and 1970s show this. Unfortunately, the enormous pressure of growing numbers of children in Egypt and the priorities followed in allocating scarce public resources has meant that the rate of increase in schooling per capita of eligibles, while still positive, has slowed down.

When young women are able to work prior to marriage, that too reinforces the formation of the actor's, as opposed to the spectator's view, and has some of the other capacity-building effects that come with schooling experience even if it is not a substitute. Depending upon the workplace, there is likely to be an encounter with new options and new images, rather than the young woman being confronted only with the sentiments, attitudes and actions available at home and in the neighborhood. The proportion of mothers in the Manshia who have had work experience prior to marriage is not large, only 5.6 percent. Daughters are doing somewhat better; the proportion of unmarried women between fifteen and twenty-five who are currently working is 8.5 percent. Even though the situation is improving, the pace is slow considering that this increase took one generation.

Fathers' education and work-place networks

For males, not only schooling but also work experience before marriage prepares them to assume responsibilities in their roles as fathers. Men's abilities to contribute to family welfare takes different forms than those of women. They bring home material goods, information, contacts with useful networks beyond the immediate neighborhood, and may provide support at home for wives to manage the home environment. Thus, men's education and their work situations affect household functioning and child health through completely different processes than women's schooling or work experiences.

Concerning the educational experience of husbands, a caution about interpretations of Figure 3-5 should be noted. Although men generally have more education than women, age for age, comparisons of husbands and wives are a different matter; one must take into account their age differences couple by couple. Husbands in Manshiet Nasser are older than their wives by eight years on average. When this difference is factored out, precise calculation shows that the average difference in years of schooling of husbands over wives is only one year.

Primary schooling in Egypt is not sex segregated. Schooling thus provides a setting where children relate to each other, and those in authority are expected to apply gender-neutral standards of achievement. In the rest of children's daily lives, gender differences are everywhere stressed. Participation by boys in schooling at an early age may encourage spousal relations later in life that are less asymmetrical in terms of power content and may make it possible to share information and ideas more readily.

Work experience is important for fathers who have the primary duty for bringing resources from the outside to their families. The occupation of the father gives him a particular status at work, a working environment, and depending upon the particular job, security of income. It also structures the nature and extent of contacts which can help him to secure goods and services for his family. These may feed into the organization of home life and contribute to the better domestic environments and thereby to better health care at home. Certainly, fathers differ in their commitments to families. When the mother is herself resourceful, more rather than less may be mobilized by the father for the family, which suggests that the separate contributions of the two parents are often not merely additive, but more than the sum of the parts.

Fathers tap into two rather different types of networks according to whether they are in public or private-sector employment. The category of public sector includes employees working for the government as well as for the many public-sector enterprises which occupy an important place in the Egyptian economy. Only about 19 percent of husbands in the Manshia are in public-sector employment, most of them at lower levels of the skill structure. A number of draftees are also included.

Private-sector employment is more common and more varied, including workshop owners, highly skilled employees in manufacturing, and a host of different specialties in the construction trade (reinforced concrete workers, masons, plasterers), as well as a sizable number of construction laborers, and unskilled labor working as carriers. There are also many men working in commerce as grocers, greengrocers or vendors for items such as food, kerosene, and notions (see above Table 3-5).

In general, public employment is more likely to bring better support to the family, apart from income, than private employment, because Egypt's public systems offer numerous welfare benefits and security. These advantages are, however, being overtaken as the income differentials to be gained from private-sector employers increase. The policy of privatization and open economy (*infitah*) is ambiguous in this regard, because the enterprises of the private sector resist the addition of benefits to their obligations and informal economic activities escape them altogether.

FOUR

Posing the Question: Why do Children Die?

Child deaths in communities like Manshiet Nasser are rarely the result of a single dramatic episode of illness. Usually they are the end point in a chain of repeated occurrences of illnesses with little time between them for adequate recovery and catch-up growth. Hence child deaths reflect life as it is lived daily in these households. These routines of domestic life, which include the practices associated with childbearing and rearing, are the very processes which also produce health. Everyday rhythms are punctuated periodically by attempts of mothers to seek special outside treatment of illness, but most of what shapes the health of their children are the activities that constitute daily life. These daily domestic activities are themsleves shaped, however, by the nature and level of resources available to households in the communities where they live. It is these resources, therefore, that constitute the ultimate determinants of child survival.

We thus begin the search for determinants of child deaths in the social resources of individual mothers and families rather than in the etiology of specific disease states which may have preceded death. The social determinants of disease and death are easily missed if one looks only at the medical causes of illness and death. It is important to move away from locating causation in a purely physiological realm and to consider the multiplicity of factors involved in the production of health. This point is well brought out by Dubois (1979:102): 'Microbial agents, disturbances in essential metabolic processes, deficiencies in growth factors or in hormones, and physiological stresses are now regarded as specific causes of disease. . . . Yet few are the cases in which it (specific etiology) has provided a complete account of the causation of disease. . . It is generally assumed that these failures are due to technical difficulties and that the causes of all diseases can and will be found in due time by bringing the big guns of science to bear on the problems. In reality, however, search for *the* cause may be a hopeless pursuit because most disease states are the indirect outcome of a constellation of circumstances rather than the direct result of single determinant factors.'

The ability to survive the first few years of life is affected by many social and environmental factors which impinge upon the individual child, beginning during pregnancy and continuing through infancy and early childhood. The questions here are: Why do some children die during these early years and others not? Can we identify characteristics of household resources and functioning that relate to observed variabilities in the survival chances of children? These questions provide the context for an examination of mothers' experiences with child deaths in the Manshia.

While the analysis that follows seeks to relate child deaths to social conditions of existence, there is also the question of the meaning of child deaths for mothers, and this plays an important role in the relationships we study. Child deaths are clearly painful experiences for mothers. Motherhood is an intrinsic component of identity as females. Furthermore, a deep attachment to the newborn develops rapidly following birth, intertwined with what the child means to the mother as well as for the sake of the child. Women's sense of self and social identity are closely linked to their reproductive activities as bearers and nurturers of children. Repeated miscarriages and child deaths threaten deeply the sense of womanhood. Just as blood of the virgin bride, *sharaf*, divides the world of girls from the world of women, successful childbearing is the realization of woman's status. The ways in which this sense of self shapes and in turn is shaped by social practices concerning childbearing and rearing are explored in later chapters where the daily struggles of mothers to protect their children against illness and death are examined in detail.

Measuring Child Survival

One general indicator of the health status of a child population is its death rate. Deaths reflect the ultimate negative consequence of ill health. Estimates of child mortality for the Manshiet Nasser settlement are made from information collected from mothers on the number of children they have ever borne and the number who subsequently died. The proportion of children ever born who have died since birth is a crude measure of the level of child mortality in the past. It remains ambiguous until demographic methods are applied to these crude measures to transform them into refined life-table estimates of the probabilities of dying between birth and different ages of childhood.[1] One such refined measure is the infant mortality rate. Another is the proportion of children that survive up to age three. We shall use the latter index most of the time.

There are at least two reasons for measuring child mortality across a wider age range than infancy alone. First, the principal threats to survival are less sharply restricted to infancy in moderate to high mortality settings.[2] The

Table 4-1. Under-3 mortality rates for children born to women married less than 15 years by residence where childbearing commenced: reference date 1980

Measures	Mothers lived in settlement since start of childbearing	All, includes children of mothers who started childbearing before moving to Manshiet Nasser
Number of women	523	663
Women with at least one birth	414	546
Children ever born	1115	1617
Children who died	183	299
Probability of dying (per 1000 births) up to age 3[a]	169	176

a. For the method of estimating probabilities, see note 1 of this chapter. The equivalent probabilities of dying up to age 5 are 186 and 194 respectively.

mortality rates of children are indeed higher at the beginning of life than at older ages but decrease to substantially lower levels after about age three. The significance of these early years and not of infancy alone is seen in several indicators of health status. Two of them are the high prevalence of undernutrition and of diarrheal disease, both of which continue into the second year of life in many Third World settings. As a result one sees elevated death rates for the second year. The practice of grouping child deaths into two segments, under one year and 1–4 completed years, also tends to obfuscate proper analysis of the forces shaping child survival. The second of these two age ranges mixes high-risk years with low-risk years. It is easy to lose sight of the health problems of children by focusing too narrowly on infancy and too broadly on the subsequent four years of life.

The second reason for preferring an index such as the proportion dying up to age three is a purely technical one. When mortality is measured with the aid of model life tables as an intermediate step in the procedure (see endnote 1), good results are obtained for survival up to age two and higher, but there is sometimes an unacceptable margin of error in the estimates of infant mortality. For these reasons, most of the analysis in this book is carried out using the index for child mortality of proportions dying between birth and age three.[3]

In order to limit the picture to conditions of survival prevailing in the recent past, the childbearing and child death experience of women who have been married less than fifteen years is analyzed. Most of these women's children were born recently. The indirect measurement of death rates refers to all of their past experience, so the approximate reference date is an average located about four years prior to the survey, namely 1980. An additional step is to limit the measurement to women who have had all their childbearing in Manshiet Nasser, thus avoiding a mixture of experience before migration to the community with the risks that are part of life in the Manshia.

Among the sample population of 663 women who had been married for less than fifteen years, 414 mothers were identified as having had at least one child and having had their entire childbearing experience in Manshiet Nasser. Altogether this subgroup of mothers had 1,115 births that were subject to the risk of subsequent death. Estimates of mortality rates for these children reflect the risks prevailing in Manshiet Nasser itself (Table 4-1).

Around 1980, 16.9 percent of children were dying before reaching age three in Manshiet Nasser, which is a moderately high level of mortality. Compared with Cairo as a whole, Manshiet Nasser's rates are on the order of 40 to 50 percent higher, for approximately the same date.[4] If the comparison could be made for similar classes of population, the difference would certainly not be as great; indeed, it might disappear. For example, we know from other studies that there is more than a two-fold difference in infant mortality rates between children of women with no education and those with a high school level of education in Cairo.[5]

A question about sex differences in infant and early childhood mortality is often introduced, because differentials imply that somewhere among all the factors that influence mortality, a bias exists in favor either of boys or girls. Estimates by sex for Manshiet Nasser suggest that male mortality is higher than female, but the difference is about what one would expect by comparison with external standards such as the 'West' model life tables of Coale and Demeny (1983). To estimate a small differential with confidence requires excellent data and a higher number of cases than were at our disposal, so the failure to detect a sex differential in mortality rates should not be taken as the last word on the subject.

Determinants of Survival Chances

The level and quality of child survival is related to the social and material conditions of the community and the households in which childbearing and rearing occurs. We have suggested that these conditions of the community be viewed as the outer layer of a system of multi-layered determinants of child survival. In this chapter we shall look at the resources which households have, and ask how various configurations of these resources are associated with differentials in child mortality. This will open many questions, because we will not, at this stage, be filling in the links that lead to child deaths as such. In later chapters we shall examine the intermediate social, nutritional, and disease processes which are these linkages and are themselves shaped in many ways by social conditions. The intermediate processes do not exist independently of social conditions which structure them.

Statistical representation of child mortality at the level of individual households

We begin by constructing a statistical model that describes our data in terms of associations between household resources and child survival. The dependent variable is an index of the 'death rate' constructed for the children of each mother individually. The procedure is from the Trussell-Preston methodology for the analysis of covariates of child mortality (1982). The child mortality index is formed by dividing the actual proportion of deaths among children ever born to a particular mother by the proportion dying that would be expected for mothers of her marriage duration in the population as a whole. The expected proportions, by five-year duration groups, are based on a model life table with a proportion dying up to age three of 168.8 per thousand births as we found above.

For the population as a whole, the mortality index averages 1.0. Particular mothers vary above and below 1.0 according to whether they have poorer or better than average experience respectively with child deaths. Those mothers who have no deaths among their children receive an index number of 0.0, whereas others range up to as high as 7.5, which is unusual. The method has gained wide favor for investigating correlates of child mortality.

Statistical representation of household resources

Several dimensions of household resources are considered as independent variables. The range of variability in each of these resources within the Manshia is somewhat limited. This constrains efforts to probe by multivariate analysis for statistically significant associations with mortality. Nevertheless, the variation among households exceeds substantially what a casual inspection of the community might suggest and is sufficient for our purposes. There are multiple variations, which yield by statistical analysis important findings concerning how children are affected by differences in the resources of the households where they are born and reared.

The previous chapter described several clusters of household resources potentially related to the welfare of the household and the health of its children. The information about these clusters will now be compressed and the clusters will be represented by statistical indicators.

The structure and functioning of the household will be represented by classifying the households in which children live into complex households, simple households, and female single-parent families living alone. There are some instances where the woman has experienced a change in living arrangements since she began childbearing, thus altering the child's rearing environment.[6] We cannot expect strict correspondence between the information on types of households at the time of the survey and conditions obtaining while the children have been at risk of survival. We make the assumption that the exceptions will not be too many to vitiate the use of the current household structure as an indicator of the child's home environment during infancy and early childhood.[7]

The next two variables refer to the human resources of the household. They are much less time-dependent; indeed, they are the endowments with which couples have begun their families following marriage.

The personal resources and abilities of the mother to transform household resources into welfare for the family will be represented by her schooling experience. This index captures directly some of what we want to include, but has to stand as a proxy for much more. Earlier discussion has pointed to the importance of schooling in a woman's formation and capacity to act effectively on behalf of her children, but we recognize that there are many other factors as well, particularly in a community where the current mothers had so few chances for schooling.[8]

The contributions of the father's personal resources to the functioning of the home are represented by his schooling experience as well, recognizing that he has been formed and acts on the basis of additional socialization experiences as well. At a second stage of the statistical analysis, information on his sector of employment, public or private, will be included to form a variable that measures some additional ways in which he has potential to contribute to the household.

Material resources of the household are represented by considering several aspects of this potentially important influence on child health and survival. One of these is income. However, a serious problem for multivariate statistical modeling is that the current income of the household is not likely to represent well either the level or the differences among households that obtained during the earlier time when children were being born and were at risk of survival. Incomes in the Manshia have changed rapidly, some types of work gaining more out of the buoyant conditions of the late 1970s and early 1980s than others. The variable for current income will be of interest in later chapters when we are looking at current health conditions of children. However, it does not seem to be appropriate when looking at risks of survival for births spread over a period of up to fifteen years in the past and centered on a date more than four years prior to the survey. Another approach is adopted.

Material conditions of the household are represented by an index of material possessions which is likely to have been more stable than current income over the years preceding the survey. One purpose of the index is to reflect, even if in a limited way, material resources available for the day to day life of the household. It has a special advantage in addition; the items we have selected are appliances directly useful in homemaking activities; thus, they can show the extent to which the household is committed to the home care of its members relative to its commitments of resources in other directions. For those who receive income there are important alternatives to support of household expenses which include acquisition of land, construction, business enterprise, personal expenses, support of kin, and education.

The material possessions include television, which is found in 79 percent of the children's households. The presence of a television set represents material conditions; and in addition it is a source of information and education useful for homemaking. The home decoration program on television is as popular among women as soap operas and Arabic films. It is watched carefully by many women who are consciously trying to learn how city people live and modernize their homes. Television is a powerful conduit of the cultural constructions of the middle classes.

Butagaz (bottled gas) cookers are substitutes for the ubiquitous primus stoves that are responsible for many accidents and are less efficient as cookers.[9] *Butagaz* cookers are found in 61 percent of the households. There is a popular Egyptian washing machine that substitutes for the woman's labor of washing clothing and bed linen in a large plastic container. It does not spin dry and is not connected to the water pipe or sewer, but reflects commitment to reducing the labor of house work. It is found in 59 percent of households. Then there is the electric fridge, found in 21 percent of households, which is valuable for food storage and handling, potentially contributing to less contaminated diets especially in a hot climate.

The value of consumer durables for the families is not limited to their express functions. These items are also viewed as signs of participation in modern urban life. One community resident observed that there are two kinds of people living in the Manshia, the *Saidi* and the 'city people.' She explained that the city people were those who knew how to look around them, see how people live in the city and were not afraid to change. Although technically she and her husband are *Saidi*, because their fathers came from Sohag, they are really city people because they are open to change.

They are urbanizing their life style. They send their daughter to school. They have bought a dining room table with six chairs, a television, and a washing machine. They have a stove with an oven, but find the bottled gas expensive and so use their primus stove as well. Next they plan to buy a color television. This family's life is certainly made easier by the appliances they possess, but the possessions also have a meaning beyond their utility and affordability.

Table 4-2. **Effects of household composition, schooling experience of the mother and father, and material possessions on child mortality rates: deaths per 1000 births up to age 3**

Grand mean of the under-3 mortality rate = 168.8

Variables	Number[a] of mothers reporting	Effects on mortality rate Gross Unadjusted	Net Adjusted	p value of the F statistic[d]
Covariate: Years mother has been married [b]	414	b	b	.004
Household composition [c]				.001
Complex household	64	+ 92.8	+ 92.8	
Female headed single-parent family living alone	23	+ 45.6	+ 40.5	
Simple household	327	- 20.3	- 20.3	
Schooling experience of mother and father: 5 years or more				.034
Neither parent	248	+ 20.3	+ 18.6	
Only mother	31	+ 5.1	- 3.4	
Only father	88	- 10.1	- 11.8	
Both parents	47	-123.2	- 97.9	
Index of material possessions				.041
Low (0 to 2 items)	229	+ 23.6	+ 21.9	
High (3 or 4 items)	185	- 25.6	- 23.6	

a. Unweighted number of observations. A weighted model is estimated. Weights are the number of children ever born normalized to the total number of mothers. Hence, the F statistics are based conservatively on the number of mothers (not children) which is appropriate when the observations of children are 'clustered' for each mother. N of children = 1115.

b. The regression coefficient for the relationship of years married to the mortality rate is + 9.28, indicating that mortality is improving over time. Net effects for the categorical variables reflect an adjustment for the effect of this continuous covariate.

c. Categories are as shown in Table 3-1. The simple households are resident couples with their unmarried children, with rare exceptions. Single-parent families are shown in a category of their own (see category 3 in Table 3-1), limited here to female parents.

d. Defined as the probability that the result is due to chance.

Note: Analysis of variance shows no statistically significant interactions among the variables. Multiple R^2=.09.

Multiple classification analysis

To estimate the separate effects of each independent variable on child mortality a suitable multivariate model needs to be selected. We will be looking for the net effects on the mortality index, which means the effects after adjusting for the influence of other variables. Multiple classification analysis (MCA) is the method selected, although we have computed other types of models as well to assure ourselves that we are not misrepresenting the data by the choice of MCA.[10] An assumption of this method is that the net effects of each independent variable on the dependent variable is the same regardless of the level of the other independent variables. While MCA is very similar to least-squares regression, the assumption of additivity distinguishes and simplifies its interpretation. This characteristic of the statistical model allows us to add the net effects together to obtain an estimate of their combined effect on the dependent variable; this characteristic of the MCA model is exploited in a section below.

The MCA model for our data is presented in Table 4-2. Some technical points may be mentioned at the outset. 'Effects on the mortality rate' are differences from the overall mortality rate that are attributable to the particular household resource or personal characteristic. The gross effects are the simple associations between one independent variable and the dependent variable (mortality rate), the same as would be found in a bi-variate analysis. The net effects are the associations after adjusting for the effects of all the other variables on the association. Usually net effects are different following adjustment, but when they remain about the same it means that the independent variables are not themselves associated with each other.

A continuous co-variate is included, namely the years the mother has been married. Its purpose is to adjust for the positive effect on mortality (higher mortality) for children born further back in time as compared with children born more recently. Child mortality is declining in Manshiet Nasser, and this is confirmed by the MCA model. The regression coeficient shows a rate of decline of 9 points on the under-three mortality rate per year.

Relationships between Configurations of Household Resources and Child Mortality

The main value of the multi-variate model is to learn whether our statements about the role of different resources in producing health are reflected in the data themselves and to assess their relative implications. The model is an economical description of relationships in the data as a whole. To interpret the model, one refers to the thinking that led to its particular formulation and returns to theorizing that goes beyond the model itself.

Household composition

Beginning with household composition, it appears that the environment of a simple household is more conducive to lower mortality for children than that of a complex household after taking other factors into account. The mortality risk for children living in complex households is higher than the average risk by 93 deaths, while the risk for those living in simple households is lower than the average by 20 deaths per thousand births. Thus, there is a differential risk of 113.1 per thousand births: 92.8 – (– 20.3) = 113.1.[11] The differential is statistically significant, indicating that there is something about living arrangements in the setting of Manshiet Nasser that makes the simple household more favorable to child survival than the complex one.

This finding raises the question of what aspects of life in the simple households facilitate better child survival. In some ways, the context of an extended household provides more, not less, material and social support, including the time of other women for domestic and childcare activities, so why are these not reflected in better, not poorer, mortality rates? Does the presence of other relatives, such as mothers-in-law, mothers, siblings, or grandparents, compromise the mother's capacity to organize and manage the rearing of her children and diffuse responsibility? Are there particular configurations of resources, household and personal, which mothers are able to turn to advantage in a complex living situation? These are questions that need to be explored later.

A small group of mothers were living as single parents in their own households with children. The mortality rates for their children are higher than the mean and have a differential from the large group of simple households of 61 points. Some of these mothers undoubtedly reared their children initially in other settings; an independent simple household was the most likely, because their present setting would be a continuation rather than the result of splitting off from a complex living arrangement. So we are probably measuring the effect on children of being reared initially in a simple household setting and subsequently in a single-parent one.

Some of these women are divorced or abandoned even though still married. Others are married with an expectation that their husband will return to reside with the family again; for example, some husbands are on long-term work contracts abroad. While this is likely to bring material benefits, that is not certain. There will be variable experiences of life at home as the dynamics of child rearing revolve around a mother who is alone without a husband present.[12] She may be under the oversight of a brother-in-law, who is often the one who handles remittances, receiving assistance from him or other relatives such as father, mother, or siblings living near at hand. There are not enough cases (twenty-three) to assign precision to the amount of the net mortality effects, but the direction of the effect can be accepted. It appears, therefore, that children whose mothers are living without a husband have better probabilities of survival if their single-parent group lives on its own rather than in a complex household. The reasons why mothers make such transitions no doubt include special factors that have, in each instance, a bearing on their children's welfare.

Schooling experience of mother and father

Rather than take the mother's and father's schooling as separate variables in Table 4-2, they are combined in a single variable that represents parental resources based on the schooling experience.[13] Education in the present context is dichotomized at only five years of schooling; yet the significance of such a difference in schooling experience is substantial. Whether only mother or only father has the schooling experience has a similar effect, either one lowering the risk of child deaths. When both have had the schooling experience, there is a synergistic effect; the two together are better than the sum of each one separately. While we had expected to find a positive influence on child survival of the parents' educational resources, the great difference between the no-education situation and the both-educated situation suggests a further question. When both parents have schooling (at least five years), does this lay the foundation for a more egalitarian relationships and closer husband–wife communication? Is, this certainly could foster a higher degree of cooperation over home matters, with children being among the beneficiaries.

Household equipment

The index of material possessions is also related to better child survival. While the number of appliances is partly a function of having an adequate flow of disposable income, it also reflects the way in which income is used. In some households, cash income is managed to achieve more material convenience and support for domestic tasks, while at the same time signaling better integration into urban culture. These homes appear to achieve better survival for their children.

The effects of different configurations of household resources

A convenient technical characteristic of the MCA model is that the effect of each factor on child mortality is additive. In Table 4-3, the effects on children of living in households with different combinations of resources is explored. It is probably unnecessary to review these examples one by one, but we would suggest that the procedure be used to estimate any other configurations that are of interest.

In statistical models, estimates at extreme values tend to be less reliable than at moderate values where there are many cases on which to base the results. The best category, shown on line 3, may stretch one's credulity, although one should keep in mind that many families achieve perfect survival for their children in Cairo. The worst category is not shown, but it would be line 5 with both parents not educated. Could mortality be that poor? The statistical analysis certainly points in that direction when there is such an unfavorable resource configuration.

Table 4-3. Combinations of household resources and their effects on child mortality: illustrations of the additivity of net effects

Under-3 mortality rates (deaths per 1000 births)

Resource configuration of the household	Start with mean	Effect of social structure	Effect of schooling	Effect of material possessions	Sum of effects
1. An 'average' household	168.8	0.0	0.0	0.0	168.8
2. Simple household with uneducated parents, but with high material possessions	168.8	- 20.3	+ 23.6	- 23.6	148.5
3. Simple household with educated parents and high material possessions	168.8	- 20.3	- 97.9	-23.6	27.0
4. Simple household, only mother educated and low material possessions	168.8	- 20.3	- 3.4	+ 21.9	167.0
5. Complex household with educated father and low material possessions	168.8	+ 92.8	- 11.8	+ 21.9	271.7
6. Complex household with educated parents and high material possessions	168.8	+ 92.8	- 97.9	-23.6	140.1
7. Single-parent family living alone, mother educated and high material possessions	168.8	+ 40.5	- 3.4	- 23.6	182.3

Father's job sector and education

The potential importance of fathers' contributions to children's survival chances is explored further by constructing a variable that represents both his schooling experience and his sector of employment.[14] The variable tries to capture the quality of the father's access to sources of information, benefits, and collegial support at the workplace, which was discussed in Chapter 3. An MCA model is constructed the same as before, except that this new variable is introduced. There are no important changes in net effects or significance for the variables already discussed, so the results for the father's job sector and education alone are reported (Table 4-4).

It seems to be beneficial, reducing mortality relative to the general mean, if fathers work in the public sector or are educated men working in the private sector. Differences by education within the public sector could not be included due to a paucity of cases. Although incomes are poor in the public sector there is special access to benefits. With increasing availability of goods and services through the private sector, however, the relative advantage of working for the state may decline over time.

Table 4-4. Effect of father's job sector, combined with education, on child mortality rates: deaths per 1000 births up to age 3

Grand mean of the under-3 mortality rate = 168.8

Variable	N[a]	Effects on mortality rate Gross Unadjusted	Net[b] Adjusted
Father's job sector and education			
Private sector, educated[c]	91	- 62.8	- 47.5
Public sector, either educated or not	79	- 27.2	- 30.6
Private sector, not educated	236	+ 28.9	+ 23.8

Statistical significance: p value of the F statistic = 0.019.

a. Unweighted observations. The model is weighted as explained in notes to Table 4-2.

b. Net effects are adjusted for years married, household composition, mother's schooling, and the index of material possessions.

c. Educated is defined as 5 or more years of schooling.

The father's educational attainment makes a large difference in child survival among those working in the private sector. This tells us that the father is able to gain more on behalf of the family in the private sector when educated. No doubt education raises him to a higher skill level and, by the status education confers, also gives a stronger hand when negotiating for benefits or 'favors.'

This concludes our statistical examination of relationships between household resources and mortality rates among children. It shows that the relationships are strong ones. They add some information, but also leave open many questions concerning how the presence or absence of particular household resources affect health, and ultimately the chances among children to survive.

FIVE

How Recurrent Infections and Undernutrition Weaken Children

Death Comes at the End of a Cumulative Process

Death in young children of the developing world is usually the end point in a cumulative process of frequent recurrent infections and/or deficient diets. Only a few diseases, such as neonatal tetanus or malaria, lead to death as the direct consequence of a discrete event of illness. In general, child survival is jeopardized as infectious episodes and nutrient deficiency interact synergistically to produce growth faltering and wasting. The process is cumulative, eroding resistance to disease. A growing body of evidence from around the world points to the significance of this chronic cycle as the basic biological mechanism producing death in the early childhood years (Scrimshaw *et al.*, 1968; Puffer and Serrano, 1973; Mata, 1978).

The previous chapter showed that deaths of young children in Manshiet Nasser are related to the social and material conditions of their households. The present chapter prepares the ground for taking this insight a step further. It looks at the process by which recurrent infections and undernutrition weaken children and heighten their susceptibility to fatal disease. Those who follow this downward path, but who survive, suffer the handicap of below-normal physiological development with permanent repercussions for their young lives. We find that this process of recurrent infection and undernutrition is initiated and maintained by factors that are deeply embedded in household behavior patterns and the material structures of life in Manshiet Nasser.

Advances in medical technology, when applied, can moderate the impact of the social and material constraints. Immunization may reduce the risk of contracting disease; transmission of infections may be controlled by insecticides; or treatments such as oral rehydration therapy (ORT) and antibiotics may increase the likelihood of recovery. However, the argument made here is that improvements in the quantity and quality of survival can only be sustained when there are positive changes in the social and material structures of life that support health.

We begin by examining the health status of Manshiet Nasser's children, and show that growth faltering is a serious problem. We ask what the mechanisms are that underlie this process, and how they are brought into play. The interaction of infectious disease with dietary patterns is investigated. As we proceed, it becomes evident that biological outcomes are intertwined with and conditioned by the environmental and social settings of the household and community.

Measuring the Health Status of Manshiet Nasser's Young Children

A good indicator of the overall health status of children is their physical growth. Whether measured in terms of attained growth at a point in time, or as change over time, physical growth is widely used to assess the level and distribution of undernutrition among children. While the term undernutrition seems to imply that inadequate food intake is the basic mechanism for deficient growth, other factors are as important: maternal health problems carry over to newborns, and children's own experiences with infections may be major contributory factors to poor health. It is important therefore to think of growth faltering as an indicator of poor health that is not specific as to cause, similar to child mortality rates when they are not specific as to cause of death. Thus, growth faltering is a non-specific indicator of health status rather than a specific indicator of dietary deficiency (Mata, 1978; Mosley and Chen, 1984).

The utility of different anthropometric indices to evaluate physical growth varies depending upon the interests of the study. In Manshiet Nasser, all children were weighed and their weight-for-age is the measure of health status used here. Weight-for-age is selected because it is a nonspecific measure of cumulative growth and hence useful in exploring a wide range of factors that have varying effects over time on the growth experience.[1]

Weights-for-age are evaluated by comparing each child's weight to the median weight expected for that age and sex group using reference growth tables. Standards have been developed based on weight-for-age of large numbers of healthy children. Thus it is possible to take a single weight measurement for children of a given age and sex and estimate approximately their level of nutrition by reference to these growth standards. We use the widely accepted standards of the U.S. National Center for Health Statistics (Centers for Disease Control, 1986).[2]

The weights of Manshiet Nasser's children are compared with the reference standard by drawing the median of the standard as a solid curve in Figures 5-1 and 5-2. The individual weights of Manshiet Nasser's children

Figure 5-1. Girls' weights by age compared with standard weight by age

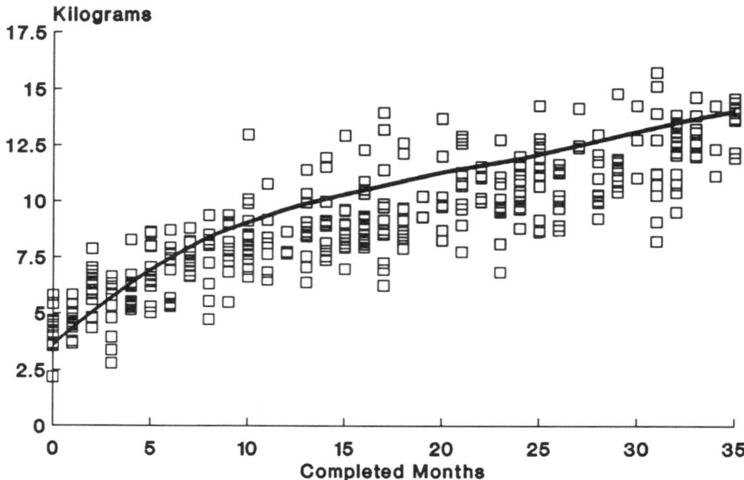

are then plotted, with small displacements whenever there are exact overlaps, so that a sense of the density of points as well as their distance from the standard is conveyed.[3]

Comparing groups rather than individuals with the standard

It is important to note that not all deviations from the standard imply problems of growth deficiency. Particular children cannot be diagnosed individually as undernourished on the basis of weight-for-age alone. Weight-for-age is

Figure 5-2. Boys' weights by age compared with standard weight by age

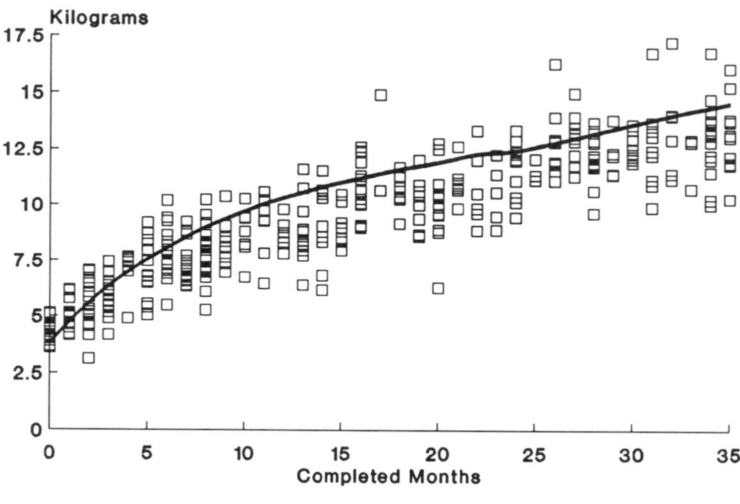

partly a consequence of birth weights, and children with varying birth weights, despite good care, may follow separate but steady growth curves with age. Normal diversity in the growth paths followed by healthy children must be taken into account when examining the individual data.

To do this, we assign standardized weight scores to each individual and then ask whether a group of children, not specific individuals, is average, above, or below the median of the reference population. The groups may be formed in various ways: girls, boys, those with educated mothers, children living in small nuclear families, children below one year of age, and so on. The procedure for comparison with the standard population is as follows.

Each individual in the study population is assigned the percentile score that he or she would receive if located in the healthy standard population; e.g., a child of eighteen months that is small for its age may be at the 40th percentile, a healthy youngster of twenty-eight months may be at the 50th percentile (median of the standard), and a heavy baby of two months at the 58th percentile. For every age, and for each sex, there is a standard to use for this computation.

We then look at children as groups of individuals. Within each group there is a scatter of percentile scores. To represent the group as a whole, we calculate its mean score. A group of normal, healthy children will have a mean percentile score of 50, which places it at the median of the reference population.[4] If below 50, the group is below the standard for a healthy population of children.

A preliminary look at Manshiet Nasser's children is undertaken by grouping the children by single months of age, first for girls and then for boys.

Figure 3-5. Education by schooling cohort, current age and sex: Percentage with 5 or more years of school

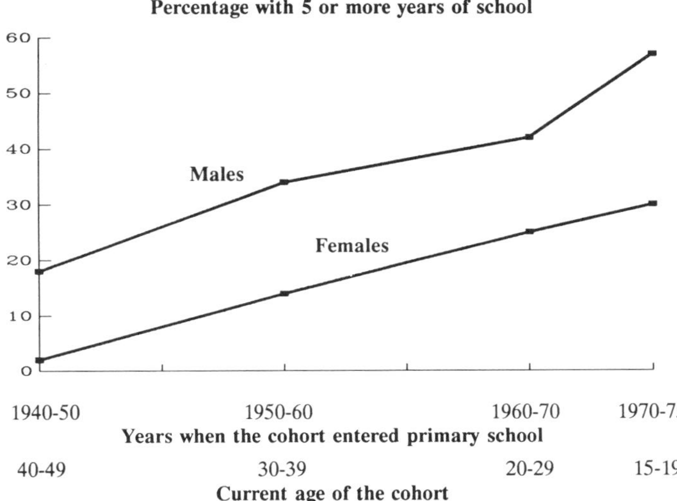

Some of the groups are small—as few as two children in one instance—so the average percentile scores are erratic and not representative at every age. To make the groups more representative, we enlarge them. This is done by making overlapping five-month groups of children centered on successive middle-month points; the first group is for 0–4 completed months which is plotted in the chart at the second month, the second group is for 1–5 completed months plotted at the third month, and so on. These procedures give Figure 5-3.

Age pattern of growth faltering

Visually, we now see two synthetic cohorts of children, one for boys and one for girls. They are 'synthetic', because they are not real cohorts observed from the moment of birth through three years of growth. Nevertheless, the demographer's practice of creating synthetic cohorts will serve us well. So long as no major changes in cohort experience are taking place, the age-specific weights can be considered representative of the weight gain (relative to the standard) that each cohort of children experiences as it passes from birth to age three. Since data are always somewhat irregular due to individual variation and measurement error, the chart should be viewed as a smooth curve as if there were no rapid advances or temporary declines at particular ages.

It is now clear that weight gain fails to keep up with the standard during the first twelve months of life (Figure 5-3). Manshiet Nasser's children start life with normal, indeed slightly above normal, weight-for-age (perinatal mortality removes some of the lowest weight cases from the data). A progressive lagging of growth sets in immediately. By about nine months of age, the children's weights have lagged so much that they are, on average, approximately at the 25th percentile of a healthy population. The curve stops its decline by the end of the first year, and then stabilizes at a level around the 25th percentile. Their undernourished state continues through the second and third years.[5] This is the period when children are most vulnerable to the risks of undernutrition. When body mass develops in this way, it means that early deficits in nutritional status are being translated into stunting that will affect the rest of life.

Comparison with other studies

This age pattern has been observed in other studies in Egypt and elsewhere in the developing world. The nationwide information on weight-for-age reported in two national surveys of nutritional status carried out by the Egyptian Nutrition Institute (1978; 1980) show a similar age pattern. The weight deficit is highest among the children in the 12–23 month age group, begins to improve in the third year and stabilizes at levels somewhat below norms in the age range 36–71 months. Children less than six months of age were not included in these two surveys.[6]

Anthropometry is making its way into more surveys, and in 1988 the Egyptian Demographic and Health Survey found the following for children aged three to thirty-six months: the proportion of children seriously undernourished, defined as more than two standard deviations below the reference population's median weight-for-age, was 13.3 percent for all of Egypt. For Upper Egypt it was 17.8 percent and for Cairo 8 to 9 percent.[7] From our own study, the proportion in Manshiet Nasser is 18.0 percent calculated for the same age range. The same reference population (NCHS/CDC) was used for both. Once again, it is confirmed that nutritional status is at its worst during the second year of life, immediately following infancy. Furthermore, the national survey showed that serious stunting (height-for-age) is prevalent—a consequence of following a growth trajectory of below-normal weight-for-age. (NPC, 1989: 182–86)

To show that Egypt is by no means unique in its age patterns of growth in early childhood, an important and influential study may be noted. The study was based on exceptionally good data collected from Guatemalan village children by following them prospectively from birth onwards for an eight-year period. It showed highly similar age patterns of undernutrition (Mata, 1978:167–201).

Are there differences in nutritional status for boys and girls?

Since our data are grouped by sex as well as age, we may ask whether there is any noticeable tendency for girls or boys to fare better. The visual impression from Figure 5-3 is that growth retardation sets in a month or so earlier for boys than girls, but leads to about the same nutritional status after the first year. Precise confirmation of this impression is obtained by computing the mean percentile scores for each sex and for the two segments of childhood, starting with the first year (Table 5-1). Girls do better than boys during the first year, but after that boys and girls are equally undernourished.

Comparing the sex pattern of undernourishment in Manshiet Nasser to national estimates of undernutrition, the latter also show no significant difference between boys and girls (1988 Egyptian Demographic and Health

Table 5-1. Children's weights by sex and broad age groups: measure is their percentile score in relation to the standard

	Mean percentile scores			Number of children		
Age group	Girls	Boys	Both sexes	Girls	Boys	Both sexes
Under one year	45.9	39.7	42.6	128	147	275
Second and third years of life	25.4	25.3	25.3	212	202	414
All three years	33.1	31.4	32.2	340	349	689

Survey). The national study represented children from 6 months (not birth) through the third year of life as a single age group. It found that the proportions seriously undernourished (more than two standard deviations below the normalized median of weight-for-age) were 13.7 and 13.1 percent for boys and girls respectively (NPC, 1989: 188).

This finding is not, however, the end of the story about differences in health by gender in Manshiet Nasser. In the next chapter we shall discuss feeding practices and the use of medical care that differ by gender of the child. Differential behavior is a signal that mothers think of boys and girls as having different needs, and believe that their care should be handled differently. Here, however, the important conclusion is that nutritional outcomes for children in Manshiet Nasser do not appear to vary by gender. This is a finding to which we shall return, because it suggests that alternative ways of meeting nutritional needs and coping with illness by gender are 'packages' of behavior which may lead to similar nutritional results.

Child survival rates for boys and girls were compared in Chapter 4. Survival for girls was slightly better than that for boys, but the extent of the difference was not significantly different from what is expected when comparisons are made to external standards. Thus, we did not detect a sex differential in mortality rates. On the other hand, differentials in mortality in favor of boys have been documented in Egypt as a whole by Batani (1982) using the 1976 census and by Makinson (1986) using the 1980 Egyptian Fertility Survey. The 1988 Egyptian Demographic and Health Survey (NPC, 1989: Table 8.8) shows a differential against males during infancy and against females after infancy. The differential against females in the 1980 EFS data was also located after infancy in the second year of life.

A possible interpretation of the national information may be suggested. Since both boys and girls enter their second year of life similarly undernourished—no sex differential in nutritional status or mortality rates during infancy—their susceptibility to repeated disease and death is about the same. However, when acute medical crises arise during the second year of life, there may be a sufficient differential in the efficacy of illness management and treatment so that girls have a marginally higher risk of death after infancy. If this is the situation, it may also exist in Manshiet Nasser and have escaped detection by our data. Mortality differentials are especially difficult to measure by sex, especially if the difference is small, unless one has both excellent data and a large number of cases.

How serious is malnutrition in Manshiet Nasser?

To the experienced eye, observing children at play on the streets and in homes in Manshiet Nasser, the youngsters appear well nourished on the whole, not at all like the children one would see in poor communities of Bangladesh, India, sub-Saharan Africa, or in many other countries. Such observations are not conclusive, however, because even the experienced eye cannot detect stunting without knowing age as well. Stunting is the typical nutritional outcome in Egyptian children who are malnourished, but nevertheless have survived their early years.

Since we have the measurements, more precise conclusions can be drawn. Malnutrition is usually scaled by categories of mild, moderate, and severe. Martorell and Ho (1984, 50) explain what happens to children as protein-energy malnutrition develops from mild to moderate to severe:

> Children cope by slowing their rate of growth and by reducing physical activity. At this stage one might observe that gains in height, weight, and other measures are less than normal. On the other hand, biochemical indicators (e.g. serum albumin) are normal and clinical signs of malnutrition are absent. At moderate degrees of protein-energy malnutrition, activity and growth rates are affected to a greater degree, and signs of wasting and perhaps some biochemical abnormalities become evident as well. At the final stage of severity, all linear growth ceases, physical activity is curtailed, body wasting is marked, and clinical signs (e.g., hair, skin, edema, etc.) are apparent.

While scientists agree on the need to separate children by such standards, there is no strong consensus in favor of a single standard. The numerical cutting points that separate one category from the other are different from one study to the next, dependent upon the purposes and statistical materials of the study. One of the basic studies in this field, carried out in Narangwal, India, showed that weight-for-age below 80 percent of the reference standard predicted higher child mortality rates, and the increase of risk was continuous as lower weights-for-age were experienced (Cited in Martorell and Ho, 1984, 59–60; originally from Kielmann and McCord, 1978). We have adopted the classification shown in Table 5-2 to array Manshiet Nasser's children against external standards. We recognize that there is no single standard with a strong consensus among scientists in support of it. The concept of grading, however, is well accepted.

In order not to exaggerate the seriousness of malnutrition in Manshiet Nasser, we will refer to children whose standardized weight-for-age is below .80 as either 'malnourished' or 'undernourished.' Further on, we shall undertake statistical analysis of the factors contributing to, or complicated by, malnutrition in Manshiet Nasser. For these analyses, the ratio of .80 will be the cutting point.

Individual children may, as we have stressed earlier, fall into a weight-for-age category that implies malnutrition, but nevertheless be healthy individuals. In Table 5-2, we show the numbers of healthy individuals that are expected to

Table 5-2. Grading nutritional status by broad age groups: measure is ratio of child's weight to median of standard

	Percent of children in each state				
Age group	Moderate/ severe malnutrition Under .80	Mild/ moderate malnutrition .80 to .89	Satisfac- tory nutrition .90 or over	All	N
First 6 months:					
Actual	10	17	73	100	143
Expected	*8*	*16*	*76*	*100*	
Second 6 months:					
Actual	25	25	50	100	132
Expected	*4*	*15*	*81*	*100*	
Second year:					
Actual	28	35	37	100	208
Expected	*3*	*14*	*83*	*100*	
Third year:					
Actual	13	29	58	100	206
Expected	*2*	*14*	*84*	*100*	
All three years					
Actual	19	28	53	100	689
Expected	*4*	*14*	*82*	*100*	

Note: *Expected* shows the proportion of children expected in a healthy population. They are not malnourished children. The norms were derived from the NCHS/CDC anthropometric growth reference standards.

be in each weight-for-age category. The comparison of 'actual' to 'expected' brings out the point that, averaging over the first six months, there is no serious malnutrition.[8] However, as the children get older, the actual numbers exceed the number expected in a healthy population in the categories that describe malnutrition. The excess is a measure of the prevalence of malnutrition.

On the basis of these comparisons, one can make such statements as, the peak for mild to moderate malnutrition is reached in the second year of life with more than twice the number of cases of low weight compared with the number expected in a healthy population. The growth trajectories ease slightly after that, but not much. Moderate to severe malnutrition follows a similar curve by age, but its prevalence is much higher than expected. In the second year, the number of cases of very low weight is seven times what would be expected in a healthy population; it is six times in the third year. Although some improvement is seen in the third year, it may be illusory because the highest risk cases have disappeared by death and are no longer in the sample for that age group.

What Determines Nutritional Status?

So far, we have been using an indicator of malnutrition which shows only whether nutrients are adequate in relation to requirements, but does not reveal much about the causes of inadequacy. We are now going to examine the factors responsible for malnutrition, first in terms of the international literature, and then for Manshiet Nasser in particular.

Evidence from many studies indicates that in Third World settings poor dietary intake and frequent infections are the main immediate causes of poor nutritional status as measured by physical growth. Concerning diet, mothers' practices with regard to breastfeeding and the timing of introduction of supplemental foods is important. So are the quality and quantity of supplements and finally of whole diets without breastmilk. These dietary practices directly influence the physical growth of their children. Concerning infection, nutritional status is strongly affected by the frequency and severity with which children experience infectious diseases.

Mechanisms that undermine nutritional status

Infectious diseases have adverse effects on metabolism and utilization of nutrients, and frequently they also accelerate nutrient loss through fever, vomiting, and excretions. For some illnesses, notably febrile ones, there is a period of anorexia, during which the child refuses food, solid food in particular. The internationally widespread practice of restricting diets as part of well-intentioned home therapy also plays a negative role, particularly in the case of diarrhea.

By interfering with intake, absorption, and retention of nutrients, infections clearly aggravate undernutrition and may also precipitate it. Repeated infections interrupt catch-up growth and do not allow the child time to be repleted from loss of nutrients.

Undernutrition, in turn, generally reduces the capacity of children to resist the consequences of infection; undernourished children are likely to experience more severe and more frequently fatal episodes of infection. Some studies have also documented a higher incidence of infections among undernourished children.[9]

When infection aggravates malnutrition or precipitates clinical malnutrition a further synergism occurs whereby infection in turn becomes more severe in the malnourished child. In social settings where infections are multiple and frequent, and diets are inadequate, the association between undernutrition and infection tends to be strong and interactive. Health impairment resulting from one is often aggravated by increased susceptibility to the other. The simultaneous presence of these two processes in poor settings results in mortality risks to children which are greater than would be expected from a simple combination of their separate effects (Scrimshaw *et al.*, 1968).

Accumulating evidence suggests that infections are at least as important as inadequate diets and may be the predominant cause of nutritional deficiency in the developing world. The infectious disease experience of young children in poor settings differs significantly from the experience of children who have good sanitary environments and medical support. Infectious episodes which are usually rare, trivial, and self-limiting have devastating cumulative consequences for survival when they are frequent, recurrent, and more severe.

The cycle is very difficult to break without altering the community and home environments that are the source of repeated exposure to infection. Underlying the heavy disease burden is the high community dosage of infectious agents maintained and transmitted by crowding, inadequate sanitation, and the behavioral factors of poor personal hygiene, food preparation and defecation habits.

In the light of these specifications of the mechanisms of interaction between diet and infectious disease internationally, we now turn to child rearing in Manshiet Nasser to see how the interactions reveal themselves in the experiences of this community's children. A single-survey study does not provide sufficiently rich statistical data to provide definitive answers to questions about the relative importance of infectious diseases and food intake in producing growth retardation. However it does provide a good assessment of the magnitude of the infectious disease burden among the children of this urban community, and that has practical implications for a strategy to improve nutritional status in early childhood. When used together with observations of family life, it also gives a good understanding of breastfeeding practices, supplementation, and weaning, which also have implications for strategies of supporting health in the community.

Major Risks: Diarrheal and Respiratory Illnesses

Illnesses were identified by asking mothers about episodes experienced by their children during the two weeks preceding the field survey. When asked, mothers talked about respiratory problems, diarrhea, eye and ear discharges, and, in response to an open-ended query, about a host of other ailments including skin eruptions,swellings in various parts of the body and fever (*sukhuna*). The last was frequently attributed to teething. Only a little more than one-fourth of children were reported to have had no ailments during the fortnight. The survey design paid particular attention to respiratory and diarrheal illnesses since these tend to dominate the morbidity and mortality of young children in poor settings.[10]

The prevalence rates point to a strikingly high burden of infectious disease among these young children. 'Prevalence' in this context means occurrence of the illness within the two-week reporting period. Summarizing the data for all children, fully 69 percent experienced at least one of these illnesses during the previous two weeks. A respiratory illness was reported

Table 5-3. Children with respiratory or diarrheal illness by sex: measure is percent reporting an illness during preceding two weeks

Illness	Percent having illness		Ratio
	Male	Female	Male/Female
Diarrheal	43	42	1.0
Respiratory	53	45	1.2
Number of children	353	343	1.03

for 49 percent of the children and diarrhea for 42 percent. The proportion of children ill with diarrhea on the day of the survey was 15 percent.[11] It is surprising that diarrheal illness occurred almost as frequently as respiratory illness, because the field survey was conducted in the months of February to April, when diarrheal illness is at its lowest seasonal level in Egypt.[12] This tells us that conditions in Manshiet Nasser are particularly favorable for transmission of diarrheal agents and for infection.

Another clue to the frequency of illnesses is seen when both diarrheal and respiratory illness occur together. Fully 22 percent of the children (all ages) were reported by their mothers to have had both illnesses during the two weeks preceding the survey.

The prevalence of the two illnesses is shown by sex in Table 5-3. Note that prevalence is not significantly different by sex of the child. This suggests that there are no differences in childcare practices that would increase the exposure of one gender more than that of the other.

During the course of growing up, the risks of having different diseases change. Table 5-4 provides the basic information needed to discuss the way in which growing up (age) alters the risks of experiencing each of these two illnesses. The highest risk period is the second half of infancy continuing into the first half of the second year (see *Diarrheal disease*). Though not shown in the table, the likelihood of experiencing both diseases during a single fortnight reaches 28 percent as they pass through the critical period of late infancy and the beginning of the second year of life.

Table 5-4. Occurrence of respiratory and diarrheal illness by age: Measure is percent of children having illness during the last 2 weeks (winter season)

Illness	Age of child (months)					
	0-5	6-11	12-17	18-23	24-29	30-35
Respiratory	54	51	48	46	45	45
Diarrheal	39	59	53	39	33	27
Number of children	147	131	118	95	107	100

Respiratory illness

A multitude of viral and bacterial agents cause respiratory illnesses. They tend to occur with nearly equal frequency during each age range shown in the table, although there is a slight decline as children grow older. The age-pattern seems to be the one usually found for lower respiratory tract infections such as pneumonia and bronchiolitis.[13]

Our investigation could not document any higher frequency of occurrence of respiratory disease for malnourished as compared with satisfactorily nourished children; hence, we are bound to conclude, tentatively at least, that poor nutritional status does not predispose children to more frequent bouts of respiratory illness in Manshiet Nasser. The consequences of respiratory illness may be more severe for those who are undernourished, however, cumulatively contributing to growth retardation, but this could not be measured directly due to the confounding statistical factors that are present. Neither could we detect a greater susceptibility to respiratory illness with particular feeding regimes; thus showing that transmission of respiratory infections is much less dependent, if affected at all, by diet or food handling than is the case with diarrheal disease.

Diarrheal disease

The frequency of diarrheal illness rises sharply after the first six months of life to a peak of 59 percent of the children, even though it is winter (Table 5-5). The rise coincides with the stage of infancy when foods other than breastmilk begin to be introduced into the diet, and then declines among older children as specific and enduring immunity to most locally prevailing agents develops. The concentration of cases during and immediately after the weaning period and a progressive decline with age after that is a distinctive feature of acute diarrheal disease in the developing world, well documented for many places (Gordon *et al.*, 1963; Scrimshaw *et al.*, 1968; Mata, 1978).

We may look closer at the reasons for this pattern of illness early in life in Manshiet Nasser. In the discussion of mechanisms of interaction above, we drew attention to the relationship between feeding patterns and the incidence and severity of infectious diseases, particularly diarrheal illness, among children growing up in poor environments. The relationship has two analytically distinct but interrelated biological components. Foods other than breastmilk may serve as vehicles of exposure to pathogens; whether they do or not depends upon the load of infectious agents in the environment and hygienic practices. Further, resistance to infection is lowered if nutritional needs that increase with age are met by foods of low nutritional value; which depends both upon affordability and feeding practices. The joint effect of these two processes is particularly strong during the weaning period; immunity acquired from the mother and the anti-infective properties of breastmilk decline, while acquired immunity to some local agents has not yet been established.

In Manshiet Nasser, we see this two-factor process affecting children's diarrheal attack rates as they live through infancy. The immunological properties of breastmilk appear to restrict attack rates that otherwise would be higher for those children who are exposed by food from sources other than breastfeeding. To see this, compare the attack rates for partial breastfeeding with those for exclusive breastfeeding during the first half-year of life; both attack rates are 37 percent of children (Table 5-5).

In the second six months, exposure to infection increases and attack rates increase correspondingly. Attacks are not limited as successfully by breastfeeding at this time; attack rates rise to 57 percent for breastfeeding children (Table 5-5). Even for exclusive breastfeeders, the safety of their regime diminishes, because they also experience rising attack rates. Some foods other than breastmilk are being given irregularly, even though the mother continues to report herself as exclusively breastfeeding. Furthermore, this is also the time when children begin to move around and put things in their mouth.

The central finding in Manshiet Nasser, confirming earlier discussion of what to expect in poor environments, is that infants who are not receiving breastmilk have significantly more frequent attacks of diarrhea. The lowest attack rates are for the wholly breastfed (42 percent); rates rise when they are given additional foods (54 percent); and become highest when the infants receive no breastmilk (69 percent). Within this last group there are children who never initiated breastfeeding at all, and for them the attack rate is very high (73 percent).

The role of diarrheal illness in weakening children becomes more serious if they are already in a susceptible state, i.e. malnourished and lagging in growth. To show this we begin by noting that higher attack rates accompany malnutrition (Table 5-6). This association is not necessarily a sign that

Table 5-5. Attack rates of diarrhea by feeding pattern and age of infant: measure is percent reporting diarrhea during preceding two weeks

Feeding pattern	First 6 months	Second 6 months	Entire 1st year
Breastfeeding	37*	57	46*
Exclusively	37*	55	42*
Partially	37*	59	54
Not Breastfeeding	67	71	69
Number of children	146	131	277

* The statistical significance of the difference from 'not breastfeeding' is $p < .05$.

Table 5-6. Association between nutritional status, diarrhea attack rates, and duration of diarrhea among children by broad age groups: measure of nutritional status is ratio of child's weight to median standard

Age and nutritional status	Number of children	Diarrhea attack rates (percent)	Median duration of diarrhea in days[a]
First year			
under .80	46	67*	7.1
.80 and over	228	45*	4.8
Second and third years			
under .80	85	44	7.1
.80 and over	328	37	4.4
All ages combined			
under .80	131	52*	7.1
.80 and over	556	40*	4.5
both under and over .80 combined	687	42	4.9

Note: Attack rates are calculated from illnesses reported for the two-week period preceding the survey.

* Statistically significant differences at $p < .02$.

a. The median duration of diarrheal episodes was calculated by constructing life-table survival functions using all observations. The differences in median duration by nutritional status were not tested for statistical significance, but would appear to be significant.

malnutrition predisposes children to attack. However, when attack rates are high, due to whatever causes, deterioration of nutritional status is reinforced by a longer duration of illness for each episode. Note the longer durations of diarrhea that children experience when they are malnourished (Table 5-6). When caught in this cumulative process, the child remains malnourished and susceptible without the benefit of 'catch-up' growth. This is the classic downward spiral. The ability of families to break the cumulative deterioration by prevention and/or treatment of diarrhea will be discussed in the next chapter.

While acute episodes of respiratory and diarrheal illness are visible threats to the health of children, another form of infection passes relatively unnoticed. These are the parasitic infections that are common in crowded environments with poor sanitation. We turn next to these infections.

Parasitic Infections that Impair Nutritional Health

Parasitic infections involve many species of worms and protozoa. They do not become evident by being a major cause of death, but do undermine health in indirect and undramatic ways. Parasitic infections commonly have chronic and endemic patterns: acquired immunity to agents is typically incomplete and slow to develop, superinfection occurs, and the usual course of infection is asymptomatic with many children being infected, but only a few showing clinical signs of disease.[14] While it is easier to see the health implications of acute infections, it is hard to assess the consequences of parasitic infections, which are likely to be non-specific, cumulative, and possibly synergistic with other infections. The effects are thought to occur largely through nutritional impairment of the human host because the parasite not only takes nutrients away but also disturbs digestive processes (Scrimshaw, 1968; Crompton *et al.*, 1984).

In order independently to confirm that parasitic infections have deleterious effects on nutritional status, with Manshiet Nasser as the case in point, it would be necessary to face complexities of data collection and confounding variables that go far beyond the means of the present type of study. The literature is clear concerning their threats to health, and is accepted. For Manshiet Nasser, then, the question is one of prevalence: how important are parasitic infections in the community? Information on prevalence serves two purposes. First, it shows whether specific parasitic illnesses are present or not. Second, the profile of parasites points to the kinds of conditions in the community that create harmful illnesses, because each form of parasite implies particular transmission routes. This second implication will be very useful when discussing community conditions and the ability through home management to maintain health.

Approach to measurement

Our aim was to gain a good understanding of the level and variety of environmental risks within the constraint of an economical sample size. Children were selected for the stool analysis from an age group old enough to be fully exposed to infection by diet and movement around the home and neighborhood. Although newborn infants living in unsanitary environments have been found to be infected with intestinal parasites from birth onwards, the prevalence of infections tends to increase in the second year of life and to persist throughout the third year.[15] We chose, therefore, to sample the third year: i.e., two-year olds. Even within that one year, our results showed an upward drift in parasitism with age. Since most of the parasites are relatively long lived in the human host and since superinfection occurs, this is precisely the pattern of increase by age which is found where sanitary conditions are poor.

A single stool sample was taken from a representative sub-sample of 112 children aged two completed years (i.e., in their third year of life).[16] The fecal samples were examined microscopically for helminth ova (cysts cast by worms) and protozoan forms (microscopic animals).[17] A complete list of all the species of parasites identified in the stools of the children is given in Table 5-7.

Table 5-7. Prevalence of intestinal parasites among 112 children aged 2 years (third year of life): measure is percent of children having the parasite. A child may have more than one parasite

With pathogenic potential		Presumed non-pathogenic	
Giardia lamblia	68	Entamoeba coli	18
Hymenolepis nana	25	Endolimax nana	11
Entamoeba histolytica	19	Entamoeba hartmanni	10
Ascaris lumbricoides	6	Blastocystis hominis	7
Enterobius vermicularis	4	Chilomastix mesnili	7
		Iodamoeba butschili	4
		Trichomonas hominis	3

Summary	
Infected by any parasite	90
Infected by any protozoan	84
Infected by any helminth	34
Infected by any parasite with pathogenic potential	86

Note: This table includes parasites for which the infective stage is cystic. The percentages refer to cases where cysts were identified in the fecal samples.

Prevalence of parasitic infection

The prevalence of parasitic infections is strikingly high among the two-year old children of this community; 86 percent of them were infected by at least one parasite that has pathogenic potential. One way to appreciate the intensity of intestinal parasitism in individual children is to note how many of the children have multiple parasitic infections (Table 5-8). Close to one-fourth of the children were found to be harboring three or more species of parasites. While only five of the twelve parasites identified may be considered as potential pathogens, the high frequency of all of the species is indicative of high transmission rates of disease by the fecal-oral route. Bacterial infections which are associated with diarrheal diseases, particularly in the summer, are also spread by this route.

The prevalence of parasitism among young children was found to be so ubiquitous in this community that we wondered what was so special about the eleven children who had no parasites out of the 112 in the sample. Statistical investigation showed that they were distinguishable from others as a group by being on average a little younger and more recently weaned from the breast. These characteristics would suggest, given the high level of community contamination and relatively long duration of parasitic infections, that it was only a matter of time before they also would be infected.

Since intestinal parasites are acquired by ingesting excreted agents, their prevalence among young children is a good indicator of two important

Table 5-8.	Multiple parasitic infections in two-year olds. Percentage having one or more species
0 species	10
1 species	36
2 species	33
3 or more species	21

aspects of home and community environments: quality of the physical arrangements for water and sewerage, and the existence or non-existence of hygienic practices that block the transmission of parasites by the fecal-oral route. In the next chapter, we explore the reasons for the high parasite prevalence and the extent to which efforts within the home could be effective in reducing it.

Child Feeding: Breastfeeding, Supplementation, and Weaning

Breastmilk is the best food for the first few months of life and most infants can meet all their growth requirements from breastmilk alone through about the age of four to six months (Jelliffe, 1968). Breastmilk is important in the earliest months of life not only because its composition is ideally suited to the nutrient needs of infants but also because it has anti-infective properties. Breastmilk reduces the ingestion of infectious agents because it is fresh and reasonably free from bacterial contamination. Furthermore, breastmilk contains a number of specific factors which contribute to the immunological defense system of the infant against infectious diseases.

The contribution of breastfeeding to child health is particularly important in settings where other products for infant feeding of similar nutrient quality and quantity are not available or are expensive. Breastfeeding is also a preferred choice when the infectious load in the environment is high and transmission of infectious agents is facilitated by housing conditions, crowding, personal hygiene, and defecation habits.

Milk alone cannot adequately supply all the nutrients that are needed beyond six months of age. Children who are not receiving supplemental foods by the ninth month are likely to show retarded growth. However, the introduction of supplemental foods into the diet of the infant brings with it the hazards of exposure to infections through contaminated foods and utensils; and it also exposes children to dietary deficiencies if the alternative or supplementary foods are not appropriate or are nutritionally inadequate. The weaning process is thus a critical period during which the interaction of infant diets and exposure to infections impinge directly on physical growth and the survival chances of children. To find out how well feeding regimes in Manshiet Nasser serve children, we asked mothers about their child feeding patterns. We then compared these patterns to pediatric recommendations and to the children's actual nutritional status.

Measurement approach for feeding patterns

For each child under the age of three, mothers were asked a number of questions about the child's current diet. The questions focused on three basic types of nutrient sources: breastmilk, external milk, and solid or semi-solid foods. Additional questions were used to describe how the child received each of the food sources. For currently breastfeeding children, this included the suckling pattern (occurrence of night feeds and practice of demand versus scheduled feedings). For those receiving external milk, the type of milk used, and the manner in which the child was fed were recorded. Composition of the diet in terms of specific non-milk food items was recorded only for children receiving solid or semi-solid foods which were either specially prepared for them or were specially selected from the adult diet.[18]

The emphasis here was on the current diets of children, for which reasonably accurate data could be obtained and tables for synthetic cohorts could be constructed. Additionally, two items of recall information were collected: the age at which solid foods and external milk were introduced for those who were currently receiving them, and the age at which breastfeeding was terminated completely for those who were not receiving breastmilk. These additional data, though not as reliable due to recall error, generally confirmed what was learned from the current-status data. The survey data were used together with information from a participant-observation study in the community to describe child feeding practices during the first years of life.[19]

Breastfeeding in Manshiet Nasser

Almost all the children in this urban community are breastfed. It is customary in Egypt among both urban and rural mothers to give sugar water to the baby from birth for one to three days and then to start nursing, and this is done in Manshiet Nasser. The cultural ideal is to breastfeed until the second birthday, but in practice the average duration of breastfeeding is less, particularly in urban areas. Estimates of the mean duration of breastfeeding among young children of Manshiet Nasser show that mothers breastfeed for variable but relatively long periods of time; the general average is almost seventeen months (Table 5-9).

Young women breastfeed for a somewhat shorter period than older women; and within an age group, educated women also breastfeed for a shorter time, but the differences are not dramatic. The same kinds of differentials are observed world-wide. Some of the women in this community describe breastfeeding as tiring and inconvenient, giving a hint that

Table 5-9. Estimated mean duration of breastfeeding in months by age and educational level of mothers

Maternal schooling	Mother's age in years		
	Under 30	30 and more	All ages
Less than 5 years	16.3	18.2	16.9
5 years or more	15.4	*	15.1
All mothers	16.1	17.8	16.6

* Too few cases to make an estimate.

Note: Estimates of the mean duration of breastfeeding are made by using the current status of breastfeeding by the age of the child and constructing a synthetic cohort from this information.

durations of breastfeeding will decline when opportunities become available to change the pattern. Even men in the community have considerable information concerning the various types and uses of powdered infant formulas. The only women who breastfeed in front of non-relatives are those who dress in Upper Egyptian style, and who may be very recent immigrants to Cairo. Considering the current differentials, there need be little concern that these trends, including a rising level of education of mothers over time, will bring young women into childbearing in the medium-term future who will breastfeed so little that it is detrimental to the health of children.

Belief in the value of breastfeeding has by no means disappeared, even in the cities, where the advertising of alternatives and examples in the upper classes might seem to put it in question. The following report is illustrative: One of the young mothers in the Manshia said she would never share breastfeeding with any other woman, as this was a custom strictly of Upper Egypt not practiced in the city. Nevertheless, she did nurse another woman's child when requested because she said there were special circumstances. This woman, a neighbor, had healthy girls but had lost all her boys. She was near menopause and afraid that she would not be able to raise a boy. When she bore a male child, she approached her neighbor who accepted to nurse the baby to guarantee its survival. Some of the relatives and friends of the woman who was nursing criticized her for jeopardizing her own child's health, but both survived.

The time-pattern of suckling is a factor which influences the breastfeeding performance of mothers and thus its impact on child health. Two aspects of this pattern are important in assuring an adequate flow of milk: the practice of demand versus scheduled feedings, and the occurrence of night feeds. Practically all mothers in Manshiet Nasser feed their children on demand. During the day babies are kept near their mothers and women wear clothes which facilitate lactation. Night feeding is also universal and it is encouraged by the custom of babies sleeping with their mothers. In view of the responsiveness of mother's breastfeeding practices to the child's demands, it was not surprising to find that mothers were generally unable to specify the frequency of daily feeds. Only 31 percent of the breastfeeding mothers were able to answer such a question and 50 percent of these indicated six or more feedings per day. The prevalent suckling pattern seems conducive to assuring good milk flow and hence to prolonged and effective breastfeeding.

The characteristics of breastfeeding examined so far—the proportions who initiate, average length, and the suckling pattern—all suggest that this component of child feeding contributes positively to the healthy growth of children. A very small group—those who never initiate breastfeeding—show the opposite relationship. The number of children in Manshiet Nasser who never receive breastmilk is only 4.5 percent. The relative risk of their being malnourished is markedly higher than for those who do breastfeed; close to eight-fold higher in the age group from birth to six months. Since failure to initiate breastfeeding is an unusual occurrence in this community, it is likely to occur only when there is a full set of reinforcing factors such as illness of the mother or the child, anxiety due to lack of emotional support for breastfeeding after delivery, or overwork and other stresses on the mother. These factors are, in themselves, also likely to jeopardize health care for the child.

A striking characteristic of the thirty-one children who were never breastfed is the high proportion that were delivered in hospital; 52 percent as compared with 18 percent for all children. Since women usually deliver at home in this community, there may have been medical problems that took the women to the hospital and some of these same problems could have interfered with their ability to breastfeed. However, that is probably a partial explanation only, because the mothers who did breastfeed reported problems during pregnancy with about the same frequency as those who did not breastfeed. More likely, the women simply did not receive support for breastfeeding at the hospital and these particular mothers did not initiate breastfeeding at all. One widely cited study of breastfeeding practices in urban settings in four countries showed that 'contacts with health services . . . were associated with shortened durations of breastfeeding or greater propensity to introduce early bottles, independent of all other background factors' (Winikoff and Castle, 1988:153). This study also makes the point that 'women using traditional birth attendants have the highest prevalence of initiation and duration of breastfeeding' (p.150). Dr. Morley has an interesting account of how crowded and impersonal maternity wards, together with separation of the child from the mother, can set up an anxiety syndrome for both the mother, whose milk flow is affected, and attending health personnel, who initiate artificial feeding rather than giving support to the mother (Morley, 1978:114).

For the other 96 percent of children who were breastfed on average for adequate durations, and who had good patterns of suckling, the clues to deterioration in their nutritional status, insofar as it is determined by feeding regimes, are to be found in the way that food supplements are introduced into the diet.

Supplementary feeding

The ways in which breastfeeding and the introduction of supplementary foods change with age is shown in Table 5-10. It is the timing of supplementation that is of primary interest here: does it start too early or too late from the point of view of current pediatric recommendations? The evidence from several studies shows that full (unsupplemented) breastfeeding contributes to better survival rates during the early months of life, particularly in poor environments without high quality sanitary and medical support (Gordon *et al.*, 1963; Plank and Milanesi, 1973; DaVanzo *et al.*, 1983).[20] Full breastfeeding is the predominant feeding mode (77 percent) in Manshiet Nasser during the first six months. This relatively favorable feeding regime is compromised to some extent by the common practice of giving children heavily sugared drinks from a very early age onward: water, rice water, tisanes of caraway, anise, mint, cumin and fenugreek, tea, and even Coca-Cola.

It needs to be noted here that we believe that mothers reported the current feeding status of their children correctly so far as regular feeding of solids or semi-solids was concerned. However, we also observed that semisolids are

Table 5-10. Children currently breastfeeding and/or receiving diet supplementation by age of child. Percent

	Child's age in months			
Feeding pattern	**First 6 months**	**Second 6 months**	**Second year**	**Third year**
Breastfeeding	90	86	44	4
Exclusively	*77*	*40*	*4*	*0*
With external milk	*8*	*9*	*0*	*0*
With food	*5*	*37*	*40*	*4*
Not Breastfeeding	10	14	56	96
External milk only	*10*	*3*	*1*	*0*
Food (with or without external milk)	*0*	*11*	*55*	*96*
All	100	100	100	100
Number of children	146	132	211	207

introduced much earlier than our data show, in the form of intermittent tastes of adult food, fed in minute quantities, usually from the finger of the mother or another adult, and as cookies and various junk foods. This is not termed 'feeding' in Arabic and so was not reported when our interviewers asked for information on feeding. This means that most children are receiving supplementary contamination but not much in the way of supplementary feeding when the mother reports that there is no supplementary 'feeding'.[21]

In this light, it seems likely that it is the antigens of breastmilk, rather than the cleanliness of the regime, that is protecting children who breastfeed in whole or part during the first half year. Recall that we found above that both regimes had approximately the same attack rates for diarrhea. Those who were not breastfeeding had higher attack rates by a substantial margin.

During the second six months of life, additional foods are essential to meet biological requirements. Yet the proportion of children receiving nothing other than milk diets (either or both breastmilk and other milk sources) is 52 percent, when it should have fallen much more. The average age at which the semi-solid or solid food begins to be regularly included in diets is the tenth month.[22] There is no difference in the mean age at which solid foods are introduced by the sex of the child. Thus, the introduction of solid foods is evidently late according to current pediatric recommendations, and this could be one of the important reasons for the decline of the growth curve, relative to the standard, seen earlier in Figure 5-3.

The transition from full breastfeeding, with the reservations noted earlier, to a supplemented diet, and finally to non-breastmilk diets, is shown in Table 5-11.

Associations between feeding patterns and nutritional status

The contribution of feeding patterns to growth retardation may be examined by considering the relationships shown in Table 5-12 as follows. Looking first at infancy, the clearest basis for comparisons is the proportion malnourished among children not breastfeeding; it is 33 percent during both the first and second six-month segments. Earlier, we emphasized that not all children who fall into a category of 'malnourished' are truly at risk, because a small

Table 5-11. Transition from full breastfeeding to supplementation and to non-breastmilk diets as age increases. Percent of children given each regime

Age of the child	First 6 months	Second 6 months	Second year	Third year
Breastfeeding only	77	40	4	0
Supplemented diets	13	46	39	4
Non-breastmilk diets	10	14	56	96

proportion of healthy children will have low weight for age relative to the standard—this is normal (see above, Table 5-2). Looking next at those who are breastfeeding, the figure of 6 percent malnourished during the first six-month segment probably refers to healthy, not malnourished, children. The proportion rises from 6 to 24 percent in the second six-month segment, which is well above the number expected in a healthy population.

The beneficial effects of breastfeeding are seen by contrasting breastfeeding with not breastfeeding. During the first six months, it is 6 versus 33 percent malnourished. Clearly, breastfeeding is a critical element in healthy growth during the first six months of life. The advantage continues into the second half of infancy as well, but is less strong because infectious illnesses are beginning to be important and they blur the advantage. One can credit the near universal practice of breastfeeding in this community for nutritional status in the first six months of life being close to what would be expected in a healthy population of children (see above Table 5-2).

By the second half of infancy the picture changes. The prevalence of undernutrition increases substantially among children who are continuing to receive breastmilk as their sole source of food, but undernutrition is markedly less than for those who are being supplemented or have gone off the breast entirely. The interesting point is to compare those who are being supplemented with those who have completed weaning; malnutrition is the same for both (30 versus 29 percent, which is not significantly different). This result

Table 5-12. Proportion of children who are undernourished by age according to their feeding patterns: Measure of undernourished is a ratio of weight to the median standard of less than 0.80. Percent of children

	Child's age				
Feeding Pattern	**First 6 months**	**Second 6 months**	**Second year**	**Third year**	**N All ages**
Breastfeeding	6	24	34	*	340
Exclusively	*8*	*17*	*	*	*168*
With supplementation	*0*	*30*	*34*	*	*172*
Not Breastfeeding	33[a]	33	24	13	346
External milk only	*36*	*	*	*	*21*
Food	*	*29*	*23*	*13*	*325*
All Children	9	25	29	13	686
Expected proportion undernourished in a healthy population[b]	8	4	3	2	
Number of children	141	132	208	205	686

* Less than 10 cases in the cell. (a) Based on only 15 cases. (b) From Table 5-2.

could be due to the inadequacy of the solid and semi-solid infant foods given either as supplements or as complete diets, but the similarity also suggests that exposure to contaminated food becomes an equally important risk for both groups: for those still receiving breastmilk the protective effect decreases, while for the others, this benefit has been removed altogether. When diarrheal attack rates were discussed above in relation to the second half of infancy, we noted that attack rates became universally higher.

In the second year of life, when the prevalence of undernutrition is greatest in general, the children who continue to be breastfed move into the higher of the two risk groups: among the 44 percent of children who continue to receive breastmilk (Table 5-11), the risk of malnourishment is 1.4 times higher than those who have been weaned; documented in Table 5-12 where the undernourished are 34 percent of breastfeeding children, but only 24 percent of non-breastfeeding children. This is an interesting finding in view of prevailing pediatric recommendations which generally advocate more, not less, breastfeeding.

Current pediatric practice is cautious, however, in that it refrains from specifying an optimum duration of breastfeeding. It is well recognized that the contribution of breastfeeding to healthy growth varies according to the age of the child as well as the context in which it is practiced. Nutritionally and immunologically its beneficial impact is strongest in the early months of life. We are able to show this for a community where the available alternatives are poor and disease exposure is high. In another community with a different setting, the relationship might not be as strong.

While a great deal of information has accumulated on the relationship of breastfeeding to survival during infancy, the effect of breastfeeding when it is prolonged into the second year of life or later has been little investigated. There appears to be a general consensus among child health specialists, however, that breastfeeding can usefully be prolonged beyond infancy because it continues to provide a source of valuable nutrients, particularly in disadvantaged settings where the alternatives are poor (Jelliffe 1968; Morley 1978; Huffman and Lamphere 1984).[23]

Elsewhere, on the basis of evidence from some rural settings, it has been suggested that the decision to stop breastfeeding is not taken in response to age but to the physical growth and general health of the child. Children who are less well nourished are nursed for longer periods (Morley 1978: 117; Mata 1978: 222–26). According to this interpretation, one may find an association between undernutrition and prolonged breastfeeding in some social settings, because children who are not growing satisfactorily, or who are sick more often, are breastfed longer. In our field work in Manshiet Nasser we were not able to confirm this interpretation, either during the in-depth observations with mothers or in the questionnaire which asked reasons for stopping breastfeeding.

An alternative interpretation may be suggested. When breastfeeding is prolonged beyond the first year, this practice may be associated with a narrow range of diet items and with less frequent feeding of supplements, which has a negative effect precisely because the child is passing through a period of rapid physical growth with high nutritional requirements. This combination produces in two- and even three-year olds a state of undernutrition while breastfeeding continues. With children who are still receiving breastmilk, mothers may not worry as much about feeding additional foods, feeling that the child is being taken care of safely. When no longer on the breast, the need for other foods is clear. Additionally, the child is perceived to be almost exclusively the responsibility of the mother until breastfeeding stops. Feeding by others introduces a more varied diet, though that too, may have problems.

From the standpoint of pediatric recommendations, the child could continue to be breastfed, possibly with nutritional advantage, but this is separate from the need for solid foods to be introduced. They must be adequate both in amount and composition and should be hygienic as well. In the specific social setting of Manshiet Nasser, it is suggested that mothers and others who may assist h er, do not in many instances recognize the child's need for adequate non-breastmilk foods until the complete shift off the breast is made.

We have examined nutritional status and seen how its two immediate determinants, infectious diseases and infant feeding regimes, are producing growth retardation, affecting many children. Next, we shall be looking at home and environmental conditions that help us to understand why infectious diseases and undernutrition should be so prevalent. We are moving layer by layer to uncover the basic social and environmental structures that determine child health in this community.

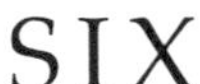

SIX

Home Management of Health and Illness

In Manshiet Nasser responsibility for children's welfare rests ultimately with their mothers, though other females, such as kin present in the household or living nearby, and neighbors, help each other in balancing housework with childcare. Fathers and even grandfathers are mobilized at critical junctures, especially when visits to doctors or hospitals need to be made. Siblings rarely make decisions of importance, though older sisters carry small children and provide a form of custodial care.[1]

Mothers fulfill their responsibilities for childcare within the boundaries of resources available to them. There are a number of constraints on their actions which are beyond their control. The structure and complexity of this division between factors within and outside maternal control is illuminated by examination of the transmission routes of the parasitic infections that were found in the previous chapter to be important in this community. As the routes of transmission for parasitic disease are identified, it is useful to keep in mind that diarrheal disease is communicated by some of the same vectors. Thus, by looking at parasites, the general system for communication of infectious disease in this community is better understood.

Transmission Routes for Parasitic Disease

The parasite survey identified five specific agents that are important in terms of pathogenicity (producing disease, or at least symptoms) which are shown in Table 5-7 of the previous chapter. These organisms have somewhat different means of transmission (Feachem *et al.*, 1983). Their relative frequencies suggest what kinds of environmental exposures are more important than others in this social and ecological setting.[2]

Giardia is highly prevalent (68 percent). It is a minute protozoan that settles in the small intestine. Giardia infection is commonly associated with chronic diarrhea and malabsorption of nutrients. It is transmitted by cysts that are excreted in the feces and may be acquired through fecally contaminated hands, food, or water. Contamination of piped water at the source of supply is another possible mechanism of transmission for Giardia cysts. They are believed to be resistant to chlorination and have been incriminated in several outbreaks in the USA and Canada (Feachem *et al.*, 1983).[3] Similar incrimination of the Cairo water supply was not seen during the period of our study, but the possibility cannot be ruled out.

Giardia may also be introduced into water that is obtained from the municipal system by handling practices in the home. All households in Manshiet Nasser store water, even when they are connected to the water network, because of frequent cutoffs. Although drinking water is stored in separate containers, these are in close proximity to other domestic water containers. For the most part, water is withdrawn from these containers by dipping, and is thus frequently subject to contamination by fecally polluted hands.

Even when drinking water containers have taps or sometimes covers, the family ingests contaminants from other unprotected containers through washing of vegetables and dishes. In addition, water containers are rarely, if ever, thoroughly cleaned.[4]

Hymenolepis nana (dwarf tapeworm) is the most frequent helminthic (worm) infection, affecting one-fourth of the two-year olds. The eggs of the adult tapeworm are infective immediately at excretion, and disease transmission can occur hand-to-mouth directly or from person to person in circumstances where facilities for hygienic excreta disposal and for washing after defecation are lacking. *Hymenolepis nana* can have a rodent as well as human host, and thus its presence may reflect rat feces in food as well as poor human hygienic habits. The most common symptoms of disease associated with this tapeworm are diarrhea and abdominal pain.

Infection by *Hymenolepis nana* is more common among children than in adults, and is particularly persistent when children are allowed to defecate around or near the house. The feces of infants and toddlers are not considered by most mothers in the Manshia to be infective so they are widely distributed. Mothers regard the soiling of their own clothing by infant urine or feces as acceptable unless they are dressed for a special occasion.

Entamoeba histolytica, *E. coli*, *E. nana*, and *E. hartmanni* together form the next largest source of infection, with 36 percent of the children harboring one or more of these parasites.[5] The prevalence of *Entamoeba histolytica* alone, which has pathogenic potential, is 19 percent. The amoeba cysts are usually spread directly person to person and by food handling, which implies inadequate hygienic practices in the home. In general, the amoeba species may be taken as a good indicator of the overall quality of domestic hygiene.

In Manshiet Nasser, the presence of amoebic infection reflects defecation habits of children, as does the presence of *H. nana* (dwarf tapeworm). Discussing the epidemiology of *E. coli*, Feachem underlines the fact that 'human feces, most probably from children . . . are the major source of infection' (Feachem *et al.* 1983: 205–206). The parasite survey also showed that children living in homes with more siblings (under age twelve) tend to have higher infection rates for *E. histolytica* (amoeba).

Adults, particularly caretakers of children and persons selling snacks or food, are also implicated in the fecal-oral transmission route. In the Manshia, a great deal of food that is consumed is prepared outside one's own home, and this reaches very young children as well. Cooked breakfast foods are more often purchased than made at home, and many mid-day meal foods are also prepared commercially. Staple foods such as white cheese and clarified butter are sold in small quantities, taken by hand from their original packaging at the grocery store, with a risk of contamination. Many of the sweets loved by children are sold in the streets, unwrapped and uncovered, and thus continuously exposed to flies.

It is widely thought that amoebic cysts, like Giardia cysts, are resistant to chlorination, and that drinking water supplies may serve as a mechanism of spread as well. The systems of water storage in households of Manshiet Nasser are thus potential transmission vectors due to the opportunities for pollution of the vessels used to store drinking water.

The next two parasites have significantly lower rates of prevalence in the Manshia, indicating that their transmission routes are less important, except that they overlap with the others.

Ascaris (roundworm), which is quite prevalent in Egypt as a whole, is less common in Manshiet Nasser (6 percent). The eggs of *ascaris* require maturation in the soil, and do best in moist and shady places. The low prevalence in Manshiet Nasser reflects the inhospitable environment of this rocky, dry and warm hillside where soil and moisture are scarce. In other circumstances, it would be a very common parasitic infection. The complete absence of infection by any hookworm species is also notable. However, they too need a period of time in moist soil for their eggs to hatch. Furthermore, hookworm is a more common infection among adults than children.

The low prevalence (4 percent) of *Enterobius vermicularis* (pinworm) may also be due to the warm and dry conditions found in the settlement, although stool surveys typically underestimate its prevalence. The eggs of this worm are usually laid around the peri-anal area and get into the bedding rather than being excreted. In Manshiet Nasser, bedding is frequently aired in the sun, which would reduce transmission of pinworms.

The specific parasites found in Manshiet Nasser, their prevalence among young children, and the high prevalence of diarrheal illness together suggest that home and community environments are very conducive to transmission of contaminated feces.

Community Factors that Sustain Disease Vectors

Very early in life infants begin to be carried from their own homes into other neighborhood environments by mothers and siblings. As toddlers, they become the neighborhood's children. Exposure to contamination from the ground, from food, and from personal contact with other people increases. Thus, the hygienic practices relevant to parasitic and diarrheal infections are not only those of the mother and other household members, but also the practices of relatives, neighbors and other children. Defecation practices, food handling, and the transport and distribution of water are major vectors that are partially within the management domain of each child's mother, but also depend upon the activities of other persons.

Thus, one must look to hygienic practices both within particular homes and in the neighborhood, the latter being a social sum of behaviors of many adults and children which have effects on each other's well being. Some households are more successful than others in maintaining household hygiene, but it is very difficult in this community to control children's exposure to contamination in public space and in the homes of others.

A few upwardly mobile families in the community make heroic efforts to keep their children inside the dwelling unit until they reach school age, in order to ensure control over exposure to various community life ways. This strategy entails tight restriction of interaction with adult members of the community, which may have a downside as well: less participation in the social support system of the community. For families living on the ground floor, control over children's movements is practically impossible. Those who live at higher levels in the increasing number of multi-story apartment buildings, may exercise more restraint on children's movements in public areas. However, the majority of children in the Manshia could never be reared in isolation from the neighborhood.

A way to appreciate the importance of the community's hygienic situation, as opposed to the specific one of the individual household, is to ask why it is that there is no significant statistical association among children with respect to the three most common parasitic infections: Giardia, *Hymenolepis nana*, and *Entamoeba histolytica*. This is probably because the living conditions and hygienic practices in this community are generally so poor, and children are so exposed outside as well as inside their homes by the specific routes of spread, that no association by species of infection is caused by factors that differ among households. The two-year-olds, for whom the parasite survey was conducted, live at risk in the community as much as they do in the differential conditions of their particular homes.[6]

Hygienic Habits

Dense living conditions, together with the lack of basic water and sanitation services, hinder learning and adoption of satisfactory personal and domestic hygienic practices within the homes. Descriptions of these practices come from in-depth observations. The following account is from our own work in Manshiet Nasser.[7]

Most of the dwelling units in Manshiet Nasser are quite small, so that rooms serve multiple purposes. Any room, including one furnished completely as a bedroom, may be used to receive guests, to prepare food, or for sleeping. In the part of the community with piped water, kitchens and bathrooms are sometimes in the same small space. These facts set the problem of maintaining cleanliness.

Housecleaning is a comprehensive undertaking which is done either in full or not at all on any given day. To clean the house means to beat all the rugs, if any, wash the floors, sweep the courtyard, put everything away, and make the beds. This is the job of adult women; neither children nor husbands participate. Once brought to the required level of cleanliness, the condition of the household is basically ignored until another comprehensive cleaning. No maintenance of the state of cleanliness has been observed in the community. On the contrary, deterioration sets in almost immediately, with men putting out cigarettes on freshly swept rugs, women often peeling vegetables onto the floor and only pushing the peels away, children scattering things without being made to put them away. Nevertheless, this state is defined as clean, as there is every intention of returning to the hygienic state after a certain interval. Where the woman does not work, the interval is generally twenty-four hours, but even where it is longer, interim measures are generally not taken.

Laundry is not part of general housecleaning. Its scheduling depends on the time of arrival of the water truck in households which purchase water. Where the household carries water, washing is done early in the morning so that women can get access to taps before crowds come. Tremendous effort is spent in getting clothes sparkling clean, and all kinds of preparations are used, including lye crystals, various types of soaps, and blueing. Many households own Egyptian-made washing machines, but much hand washing is nonetheless entailed. Clothes are dried on lines from windows, balconies, and in the yard. When dust or industrial pollution is heavy, they are turned inside-out while drying.

No effort is made once the clothes have been put on to keep them clean, and the clothing of women in particular is often dirty. Men whose work soils their clothes dress in old, often ragged clothing during the day, or use their pajamas, but when the work is finished they change into new, 'good' clothing. Women do not change clothes during the day unless they are leaving the community. Girls of marriageable age often change their clothing several times a day.

Disposal of gray water is a problem for households that lack working sewerage connections, especially on laundry days, when large amounts must be gotten rid of. Stringent rules govern disposal. Prior to the institution of the solid waste collection service in the community, the water was carried to vacant lots in tins which also contained the garbage; this involved considerable effort, as it meant going to the perimeter of the community. Now that solid household wastes are removed by the Zabbaleen, women dispose of water onto the streets. Densities are high, however, and indiscriminate water disposal would quickly produce mud holes in the roads. The rules call for a woman to scatter the water which she is disposing over as wide a surface as possible, though she need not go outside the area directly in front of her house, and not to dispose of a great quantity of water at one time. If she does several loads of washing, she should dispose of the dirty water gradually, so that the first lot has a chance to dry before the second is thrown. If she is careless, she is shouted at by her neighbors.

Keeping clean is certainly a labor-intensive process. Households where a son has married and brought the new wife to the household have, in some observed instances, experienced an improvement in household hygiene, which can be attributed to the larger labor force that becomes available. However, this is temporary, since the arrival of more babies takes increasing amounts of labor time and questions of who is responsible for childcare and general hygiene of the home can become diffused.

Another area in which discipline is firmly enforced, and children are pushed to conform to adult standards, is in eating from a common plate. Meals are served on large aluminum trays on the floor, or on a low round table (*tabliya*); each item is on a separate plate, but there are no empty plates for the diners, and no forks or spoons. Small pieces of bread are used for picking up cheese, eggs, or cooked food, the last of which is most often prepared in a sauce. No child is asked to wash hands before eating, nor does any adult do so, but each person is expected to take food from the part of the plate which is directly in front, all eating toward the middle, and children are carefully watched to make sure they do so, even quite small children. Bearing in mind that weaning is accomplished by moving children from breastmilk to family foods without much intermediary provision of special diets, these practices have mixed hygienic effects, some helpful and some not in protecting child health.

The Interaction of Physical Infrastructure with Hygienic Practices

When assessing the factors that elevate exposure to infectious diseases, it is useful to distinguish between rules of conduct that pertain to standards of personal and household hygiene and physical conditions in the home that may increase direct exposure to pathogens. In every culture there are rules of behavior that derive their meaning from popular wisdom that indicates what is important for maintenance of health. These rules of conduct evolve under specific physical and social conditions and may lose their usefulness as these conditions change. In discussing the idea that there is more to environmental sanitation than 'technical plumbing,' Dubois (1979:132) makes the important observation that: 'Hygiene involves a social philosophy that must take into consideration the human and economic aspects of the cultural pattern for which it is designed.' Therefore while hygienic practices and physical conditions are analytically distinct factors influencing risks of contracting disease, in practice they are closely intertwined.

Where water supply and waste disposal are deficient, the sanitary discipline necessary to minimize the risks of exposure places enormous daily burdens on household members. We made an estimate of the effort required when water is taken from storage containers and waste-water disposal is lacking. To wash hands with soap needs a second person to pour the water over them and a basin of water to be disposed of subsequently. Adult labor to do this for children after each defecation and before taking food, including snacks, as well as to clean themselves after handling diapers and their own washing-up needs, is surprisingly demanding. At a minimum, thirty hand-washing operations per day for mother and her children is our calculation, all of them requiring pouring and disposal of waste water as well. Allow three minutes for each operation, and the total is about one and a half hours per day, most of it demanding the time and oversight of a busy mother.

Although 24 percent of households had water taps in their dwelling units or elsewhere in the building, only 18 percent had both water taps and a sewerage connection with which to dispose of waste water. This was in 1984 when the settlement was over twenty years old and much increased in size. By 1990, we estimate without benefit of a survey that the situation has improved, with perhaps one-half of households now having access to piped water in the dwelling or building. Water storage continues, because the tap is at a distance or the supply is not continuous. Sewerage connections are now more prevalent, with perhaps one-half of buildings connected. Faults with the connections are still a serious problem, needing frequent repair or being left out of order.

The relationship of the incidence of disease to household physical environment is well documented (Moore *et al.*, 1965; Esrey *et al.*, 1985). It is not difficult to understand how diarrheal diseases in particular, which are spread by the fecal-oral route, are more likely to be transmitted in families that have only a limited supply of water for washing and no proper disposal facilities. The availability of good sanitary infrastructure in the household does not guarantee, but may facilitate, good hygienic behavior. We decided to check on two of these relationships.

Soap and water

During the course of the household visits the interviewers observed whether soap was available for hand washing somewhere in or near the latrine facilities. The presence of soap is a good indicator, although admittedly an imperfect one, of the propensity to wash after defecation. The impact of hand washing, particularly after defecation, on the spread of many agents of diarrheal disease is well recognized.[8] Another reason for collecting this information is that the presence of soap is correlated with domestic hygienic practices in general serving as an indicator when the details of hygienic behavior cannot be surveyed home by home.

Overall, only 12 percent of the households had soap available near the toilet at the time of the survey. Soap can improve the hygienic quality of daily

Table 6-1. Factors influencing the availability of soap in households with children who are less than 3 years old

Variables (reference category shown in parentheses)	Means	Coef-ficient	Relative risk	P value
Dependent				
Soap available in household (No) Yes	.12			
Independent				
Sanitation (incomplete or none) Both piped water and sewer	.17	1.221	3.4	.001
Mother's schooling (less than 5) 5 years or more	.20	.988	2.7	.001
Household income per month in tens of Egyptian pounds (continuous variable)	16.43	.016	2[a]	.079
Statistics				
Likelihood ratio	44.780			
Chi-square probability	0.001			
Number of children	697			

Notes: Multivariate logistic regression. For the categorical 0/1 variables (reference category shown in parentheses), the mean shows the proportion having a positive response. When the slope coefficients are positive they indicate better nutritional status relative to the reference category.

a. As this is a continuous variable, the statistic shows that a change in one unit of household income (LE 10) changes the probability of having soap by 2 percent.

life, yet it is persons with abundant water and disposal facilities who are more likely to use it. We examined this point with statistical modeling for the households with young children in them. Those that have both piped water and sewer connections either in the home or in the building are 3.4 times more likely to have soap available in or near the toilets (Table 6-1).

A logistic regression was used in which water and sewerage are taken together as a single independent variable, not separately, because sanitary effectiveness depends upon their working together. The two additional aspects of the household context, mother's schooling and household income, are included in order to examine the influence of these resources on having soap present. The household's chance of having good water and sewerage depends more on the location of the dwelling (hookups are necessary) than on its own income and other household resources. Therefore, we can include these household variables along with the sanitary situation in the same model, considering them to be relatively independent variables determining the soap outcome.

While the presence of educated mothers and good sanitation both contribute significantly to increasing the use of soap in the home, it is sanitation that has the major effect. This indicates that the use of soap is more prevalent where it is more practical. The finding is an important one, as it shows clearly that physical infrastructure promotes health by facilitating good hygienic practices.

The importance of soap and washing up in the transmission of excreta-related pathogens is underlined by another of our findings. This one comes from the parasite study. Where soap is available near the latrine, rates of infection by *Hymenolepis nana* (dwarf tapeworm) are significantly lower. Probably the reason is that this parasite is commonly transmitted directly hand to mouth and less through food or water.

Diarrheal prevalence and sanitation

Further support for the strategic role of sanitation infrastructure comes from examining children's experience with diarrheal illness. Diarrheal attack rates among those children living in homes with both water and sewer connections (located either in the home itself or in the building) were lower by 22 percent than in households without these facilities. This suggests that water and sanitation do make a difference, whether the control over transmission of infectious agents is achieved with the aid of soap or by means of other hygienic practices. While the level of statistical confirmation is not high for the sanitation variable ($p=.11$), the direction of the effect is consistent with the argument we have been making.[9]

Nutritional status and sanitation

Another way to see the deleterious effects of poor sanitation is to look at the nutritional outcome for children when they go off the breast as compared with those who continue. Presumably they are protected from environmental contamination while still breastfeeding. Although children could, in principle, continue to be protected by strict hygienic practices when off the breast, this does not appear to be happening.

The growth implications of interaction of physical environment with the feeding regime, as mediated by hygienic practices, was examined statistically for infants. We found that weights were approximately the same whether there was sanitation or not for those who were breastfeeding. However, for those no longer breastfeeding, households with adequate home sanitation are able to achieve 26 percent better standardized weights for their infants than those households without these facilities (measured at the mean).[10] Thus, where domestic sanitary arrangements facilitate hygienic practices, which limit the amount of diarrheal disease, weaning to a diet of non-breastmilk fluids and solids during infancy need not be associated with growth retardation.

There is also a community-level factor to consider. The full health benefits of water and sewer connections are not achievable simply at the level of the individual household. Rather, a high proportion of households need to be equipped with infrastructure and to be implementing good hygienic practices if a mother's diligence is to bring down sharply the prevalence of parasites and frequency of diarrheal illness. That point has yet to be reached in the Manshia.

Feeding Children Beyond Mother's Milk

Our in-depth observations led us to conclude, tentatively and without benefit of precise and detailed food measurements, that the diets of children, other than breastmilk, are poor. The diets of their parents, on the other hand, are quite good. Family meals are constrained by incomes, so that the quantities of meat and poultry may be small, but a considerable variety and large quantities of cheese, fruits and vegetables are consumed. Children receive only half a cup of milk, mixed with tea, once they have made an adjustment to solid food, and they eat large amounts of junk foods.

Even the smallest child is given money to spend at the grocery, and there is no supervision of their spending. In Arabic it is called 'giving money to waste.' Favorite foods include Karate (puffed cheese snacks), cookies, and penny candies. Those who have more money to spend buy Coke. People rise early, so by the time the father arrives home at 2 P.M. or so for the main family meal, the children are likely to have eaten many snacks, and are not hungry, so they miss the meal. Later in the day they are hungry again, and again snack.

Weaning to solid foods is by preference for items which the child can hold itself. The first foods, then, are also items like Karate and cookies, given to the child on demand and as a treat. There is no idea that these foods may not be nutritious; on the contrary, the extensive television advertising of these items has established a consuming community which sees them as modern and good. Children watch television and see new things advertised, demanding them at groceries until they make an appearance. The normal family diet is not withheld by any means from these children, but there is no insistence that they partake if they are not hungry, or that they avoid filling up with other foods before the meal. On the contrary, many mothers on limited budgets push their children to eat filling snack foods so that they will not insist on more later in the day, a strategy which is likely also to depress the appetite for lunch.

The impression that children who have stopped breastfeeding are uniformly receiving poor diets would not be correct. There is evidence of variability. Among children who are no longer breastfeeding, those who live in simple household formations with better income and educated mothers, maintain better weights than the other children. While this evidence is not a direct measurement of the diet—the survey could not collect nutrient details on solid food diets of children and adults—it suggests that these mothers are likely to be providing better child feeding.[11]

Care During Pregnancy and Childbirth

It is increasingly recognized that the maintenance of child health begins very early, physiologically, emotionally, and psychologically, with the reproductive health of the mother. The health she sustains during pregnancy, delivery, and post partum is critical for the newborn's health and development thereafter. Reproductive health of the mother may be seen, therefore, as a single concern with twin outcomes: the mother's own welfare and that of her children, particularly at the start of life.

In Manshiet Nasser, the state of pregnancy is intensely desired, not only for the first child but for subsequent ones as well. The women take pride in their competence in childbearing, making a linguistic distinction between the woman who has more than one child and the woman who is still *bikriya*, that is the mother of only one child. Significantly, *bikriya* is defined as having only one living child, or when applied to the child, the first child to survive. Pregnancy and even delivery, are viewed as normal events which do not require particular precautions, either medical or ritual. The idea of prenatal care is not rejected after consideration; it does not occur to most woman as relevant. Thus the mother will notify the *daya* (lay midwife) of her impending delivery, but she seeks no other contacts with medical personnel. *Dayas* are not considered to be medical practitioners, or even substitutes for medical practitioners; rather, the doctor, under some circumstances, is seen as a substitute for the *daya*.

Abnormal pregnancies (defined as situations requiring medical care) arise, but whether a doctor is consulted or not depends upon the woman's perception of the degree of threat involved. The need for treatment must compete with standards of modesty, as these women have never had full physical examinations, and are enjoined from an early age never to expose their bodies to a male other than the husband. If a situation is perceived as genuinely life-threatening, the injunction can be overridden, but not for conventional prenatal care. The same attitude is seen for problems of infertility. In neither case is the problem one of attitude toward the medical establishment, as these women use doctors and hospitals extensively. Since female obstetricians are rare and an appropriate female environment seldom available, only the most serious perceived threats receive attention. Prenatal tetanus shots could be accepted, but not full examination.

These views of women and their behaviors are reflected in the data we collected concerning the woman's care of herself during pregnancy and delivery for each child in the study. An examination or consultation of some kind was done in 40 percent of the pregnancies, more than half of them in private clinics of physicians. Recall was too poor for us to learn about the extent of tetanus immunizations. Indeed, they did not consult in most cases for prevention, but for problems. They visited medical personnel in most cases because a problem was perceived; 74 percent had specific problems in mind. The educated mothers (schooling of five years or more) reported more specific complaints than the uneducated, thus exhibiting greater awareness, and their use of medical personnel was higher.

At the time of delivery, the preference was clearly for *dayas*, who attended 63 percent of the births, and 80 percent of all deliveries were home deliveries (the woman's own home or that of a relative/friend). Physicians assisted deliveries in 22 percent of the cases, nurses and *hakims* 6 percent, while the rest were assisted by relatives, neighbors, or no one.

One sees reflected in the actions of mothers their definition of and confidence in what they perceive to be natural processes. Nevertheless, they do reach out to the medical system when threats to the natural unfolding of pregnancy or great anxiety are felt. These constructions of normality, threats, and needs for consultation begin with pregnancy and carry through delivery to the postpartum period. The mother's initiation of breastfeeding and care of the child reflects similar constructions with regard to her newborn. If a problem is perceived, it calls first of all for consultation with women one trusts and then with medical personnel if the problem becomes so defined. The notion of medical monitoring and preventive care scarcely exists for either normal pregnancy or early infant care.

Caring for Sick Children

Child rearing in Manshiet Nasser entails coping with frequent illness. Acute attacks of diarrheal and respiratory illnesses are interspersed with childhood diseases such as measles, whooping cough, fevers, and eye, ear, and skin infections. While sickness care has little direct effect on incidence of disease, good medical care, including advice on home management, contributes to a faster and better state of recovery and to less fatality. Without timely and appropriate care, a child's nutritional state often deteriorates and even if he recovers from a specific episode, the increased risk of subsequent severe illness, particularly diarrheal, continues for many months.

Feeding regimes during illness

Children need to continue to receive an adequate amount of nourishment during illness. Diarrhea makes a particularly important demand on mothers for timely management so that nutrients continue to be ingested and there is adequate absorption of fluid to avoid or reverse dehydration. Current pediatric recommendations stress the importance of continuing to breastfeed during diarrhea if that was part of the regime preceding illness. In the Manshia, we found women withholding solids from children who were partially weaned, saying that it was on 'doctor's orders', but we never saw a mother refuse the breast to a child with diarrhea. These specific observations are roughly confirmed by the survey.

Mothers of breastfed children with diarrhea reported in 11 percent of cases that they gave less milk, most often giving as a reason food intolerance on the part of the child. Their reduction of feeding was more severe for other items such as solid or semi-solid foods (37 percent) and external milk (63 percent). The last figure reflects the response that most mothers have who are giving milk from non-breastmilk sources by bottle or spoon. They replace this source of milk by tisanes. Since these babies are mostly not completely weaned, the modification of diet is especially unfortunate; although fluid intakes may be sustained, nutrients are not.

The subject of nutrition during diarrhea has received a great deal of attention in Egypt as a follow-up to campaigns during the mid-1980s for use of rehydration solutions to treat diarrhea. It was realized that more than rehydration was necessary to put children back on their feet. In Manshiet Nasser at the beginning of the 1990s many mothers know the recommendations for use of rehydration solutions well, but they regard them as one more among many options that they can consider. Home treatment is a very labor-intensive procedure which has to be sustained longer than most understand it should be. Furthermore, its potential value is often diminished by recommendations from medical practitioners to take medications at the same time.[12]

Seeking help for sick children

Faced with a variety of child illnesses, mothers try to piece together information from different sources in an on-going effort to formulate explanations and treatments for the conditions. Some illnesses, such as measles, are considered to be an inevitable part of growing up. Others, such as diarrhea, may be attributed to living in a 'popular quarter,' and its specific occurrences viewed as almost random events stemming from this basic fact. Whatever the nature of explanations that mothers are able to work out for these conditions, the search for treatment of their consequences goes on.

To the extent that an episode of illness is seen as serious or life-threatening, mothers seek medical treatment. This is well illustrated by the close association between perceived clinical severity of diarrheal disease, indicated by the nature of symptoms reported by mothers, and their efforts to seek medical help. For cases involving diarrhea alone, 35 percent of the mothers sought professional help, whereas when additional clinical signs, such as fever, vomiting, or blood were present, the proportion increased to 65 percent.

For less serious cases, home remedies are considered to be sufficient. Drugs and prescriptions obtained during similar episodes in the past may be used, together with home remedies involving special handling of sick children and changes in their diets. There is considerable shopping around for efficacious treatment and mothers are quite prepared to alter the course of treatment and follow multiple remedies simultaneously in an effort to bring about a cure. The search includes consulting not merely different types of sources but also various individuals with the same credentials in an attempt to hedge one's bets in an uncertain situation.

If the desired results are not produced, and if an ailment is serious, sick children may be taken to Tanta in the Delta, to the area around the mosque of Sayyid al-Badawi, a mystical center where many sheikhs are in residence (this is also the location of choice for female circumcision if the family has enough time and money to spare). Alternatively, if family resources are limited, or if the case is less urgent, they may be taken to one or another saint's tomb in the adjacent cemetery area, also for treatment by a sheikh.

It is clear from the data of the survey and from observations in the community that modern medical care and medicines are highly valued, although seldom to the exclusion of home remedies or advice from lay persons. What is of particular interest in this situation is that while the formal medical care system is regarded as highly efficacious, the encounters with it are viewed as intimidating by the families. Parents typically neither ask nor expect to receive information about the condition of their child from doctors, only instructions and these mostly in the form of written prescriptions. People believe that doctors speak a secret language which nobody outside the medical profession can understand, and that they use this language to communicate with one another in front of parents concerning prognosis.[13] They even believe that doctors often know whether the child is going to live or die, but not how to alter the prognosis. These opinions of the residents are perceptive comments on the social distance that is maintained by the medical profession, and the profession's concept of its responsibilities toward patients.

One consequence of this type of relationship is that the encounters fail to strengthen the capacity of mothers to care for their children. Their dependence on the medical system is increased, rather than their independent capacity for promoting health and cooperating in the treatment of illness. The patterns of illness care described below need to be interpreted with these considerations in mind.

Among 630 cases of illness reported by mothers for a two-week period before the survey, over half were taken for consultation to a physician, hospital, health center or a pharmacist (Table 6-2). The nature of the illness, whether diarrheal or respiratory, did not make a difference in the effort to seek help from a health professional. Although the overall effort to obtain medical attention is similar whether the illness is diarrheal or respiratory, the

Table 6-2. Professional sources consulted for treatment of diarrheal and respiratory illnesses. Percent of all cases

Sources	Diarrheal		Respiratory		All Cases	
Physician	36		39		38	
In settlement		*29*		*31*		*30*
Outside		*7*		*9*		*8*
Hospital	15		13		14	
Out-patient		*10*		*10*		*11*
In-patient		*4*		*3*		*3*
Health center	1		2		2	
Pharmacist	5		3		4	
No professional source consulted[a]	45		46		46	
All consultations[b]	104		103		104	
Number of cases	294		336		630	

a. Also included are father, a relative, or a friend.

b. Percentages add to more than 100, because more than one professional source was consulted in 7 diarrheal and 11 respiratory cases. Rounding of the subcategories gives the appearance of inconsistency with the total which is, nevertheless, a correct total including the cases of multiple consultations.

Table 6-3. Proportions of diarrheal and respiratory illnesses (percent) receiving professional consultation by age and sex of child

	Diarrheal			Respiratory		
Age in months	**M**	**F**	**Both**	**M**	**F**	**Both**
0-11	70	58	64	58	52	55
12-35	49	46	47	48	55	52
All ages	59	51	55	53	54	53
Number ill	151	143	294	183	153	336

Note: Cases are classified as receiving professional consultation when a doctor, hospital, health center or pharmacist was seen during the illness.

age of the ill child seems to affect the decision to seek treatment in the case of diarrhea. When the illness is diarrheal, there is a stronger propensity to take infants for treatment than older children, and this age pattern is particularly marked in the case of male infants (Table 6-3).[14] More attention to infants is due to the rapidity with which diarrheal disease can become life-threatening among the very young. Although the number of cases is small, the data (not shown here) also indicate that a higher proportion of both male and female infants were hospitalized during the course of diarrheal treatment as compared to older children.

Differences in care for boys and girls

An interesting insight into the subtle ways in which sex differences in childcare occur emerges from a more detailed examination of the relationship between the severity of illness and the effort to obtain medical attention. When the diarrheal episode was complicated and thus likely to be perceived as severe, mothers sought professional care equally for boys and girls. The behavior was quite different, however, when diarrhea was a simple episode of loose stools, in which case mothers tended to seek professional care twice as often for boys as for girls (Table 6-4).

We also noted that there is a greater expenditure of effort and financial resources for treatment of boys than for girls. This is implied by greater use of doctors and hospitals outside the settlement for boys (see Table 6-5 below). It appears that sex selectivity in the provision of sickness care to young children works through both the choice of whether to seek medical attention and the selection of sources for consultation.[15]

This finding on the willingness of mothers to seek medical attention more for boys than for girls for simple diarrheas is consistent with the evidence on attendance at hospitals and rehydration clinics: hospital-based studies often report that male children are brought to hospital more often than female

Table 6-4. Sex differences in treatment of diarrheal illness. Percent

Occurrence and treatment	Sex of child		Ratio of male to female
	Male	Female	
Complicated Diarrhea			
Proportion of children with occurrence	29	28	1.04
Proportion of cases consulting professional persons	64	65	.98
Simple Diarrhea			
Proportion of children with occurrence	14	13	1.08
Proportion of cases consulting professional persons	48	22	2.18
Number of children	353	344	1.03

Note: The term 'complicated' diarrhea refers to the reported presence of one or more clinical symptoms, such as vomiting, fever, or mucus, in addition to loose stools.

children and that female children are significantly more ill than male children when they are brought for treatment (UDD, 1982; Makinson, 1986).[16]

The following anecdote is quoted to show how mothers are sometimes motivated to handle boys compared with girls (Hoodfar, 1986:66-67).

> The young daughter, who had just started to walk, became ill with diarrhea, supposedly because she was teething. At the time I talked to Umm Mohammed, the daughter had been ill for four months. Her mother and others often comment on her obvious regressive growth, but she has been taken to a public hospital only once. During the same time period her elder brother was taken to private doctor and hospital for reasons of diarrhea, spots, fever and general weakness. When I tried to make the mother conscious of her preferential treatment of the son, she said, 'I know that it is only because he is older and because he is his father's son. When anything happens to him, his father holds me responsible and claims that I am not looking after his son properly. He won't stop nagging that I am not a good wife or mother. So in order to save my own skin, as soon as anything happens, I take him to see the doctor even when it is absolutely unnecessary. My husband gives me money for his son's medical costs much more willingly. Because I don't want arguments, I have to take our daughter to the public hospital, which is cheap but not very useful at all. I give her home remedies and she is all right.'

Earlier we reported that nutritional outcomes for children in Manshiet Nasser do not appear to depend upon their gender. Although mother's manage the needs of boys and girls differently when they are ill, the implication of our earlier finding is that the end results are not significantly different so far as health status is concerned.

Medical consultation

Children are taken to private clinics, health centers, and hospitals all over the city for treatment (Table 6-5). In 1984 there was only one small government health unit in Manshiet Nasser itself. It was rarely mentioned as a source of service by mothers who reported medical consultation. Many doctors held regular clinic hours within the settlement, but none lived there.

As the settlement grows, the demand for medical services also grows. There is no shortage of physicians in Egypt; their rate of graduation has created a surplus, with one of the highest physician/population ratios in the developing world and a particularly high ratio in Cairo. Since 1984, demand has drawn increased supply into the settlement. Many more evening clinics and pharmacies as well are now seen. As noted earlier in Chapter 2, the government has responded to Manshiet Nasser's political connections and additional public health services have also been opened, but with continuing complaints from the residents.

In 1984, the families were able to meet about 60 percent of their needs for medical attention for children from sources within Manshiet Nasser. They tended to seek medical help from sources outside the settlement more for infants than for older children. Again, this shows that whenever there was more anxiety, which is an age-related response, they would reach outside the immediate community for help.

Table 6-5. Distribution of visits to different professional sources by sex and age of ill children: diarrheal and respiratory cases combined. Percent

	Sex of child		Age in months		
Sources of consultation	**Male**	**Female**	**0-11**	**12-35**	**All ages**
Physician	66	67	63	69	66
Inside settlement	*50*	*56*	*48*	*56*	*42*
Outside	*16*	*11*	*15*	*13*	*14*
Hospital	27	20	28	21	24
Health center, pharmacist	7	13	9	10	10
All professional sources	100	100	100	100	100
Number of visits	203	158	176	185	361

Sickness care practices of mothers are usually considered to be related to their levels of awareness and skills, as well as financial resources, particularly when these involve seeking medical help. Among the families in Manshiet Nasser, however, neither the level of mother's education nor the level of household income could be shown statistically to have differential effects on whether professional consultation is sought at the time of illness.

One aspect of household life did appear to influence the extent to which children were taken for treatment, and that is family structure. The mothers living in simple households with only husbands and children tended to reach out for treatment more often than those living in other types of households, which is seen clearly for diarrheal illness (58 percent compared with 41 percent).[17] This finding accords well with an expectation that mothers who are the sole source of female authority in a household are likely to shape their strategies for coping with illness somewhat differently from other mothers. With greater responsibility, less emotional support, and less treatment advice from within the home, they may have greater anxiety about illnesses and their consequences. One of the means of lessening the burden of that responsibility is to seek professional consultation more often. As noted earlier, the mother also consults with nearby relations and neighbors, but they could not be held accountable in the same sense, in general or to her husband in particular.

SEVEN

The Multi-Layered Process of Producing Health

From the beginning of this book, we have used a certain metaphor to organize our inquiry concerning how families of the new neighborhoods of Cairo attain particular levels of health for their infants and young children in the course of their daily lives. This is the multi-layered process of producing health. The context for this process is the community and its households. The intermediate processes are those of child feeding, hygiene, disease vectors, experiences with illness, and therapy. The health outcomes are those of nutritional status and mortality rates for children. Schematically, we have:

Context >>	**Intermediate Processes >>**	**Health Outcomes**
Community	Child feeding, hygiene,	Nutritional status
Households	disease vectors,	Mortality rates
	illnesses, therapy	

The approach was to unfold and investigate the layers one by one, keeping in mind, however, that backward as well as forward linkages exist. Now we want to move toward a more wholistic view. To do this, we will retrieve some of the main strands of the inquiry and weave them together.

Firstly, recall that in Chapter 4 the associations between household resources and child death rates were examined. Nutritional status is antecedent to mortality since, as argued earlier, death comes to infants and young children primarily as a consequence of cumulative deterioration of health rather than as a result of specific episodes of critical illness. As in Chapter 4, the relationship of resources mobilized by the household to health outcome could be shown again, but in this instance in relation to nutritional status. This is one more way to tie together layers that are situated at either end of the multi-layered process.

Secondly, the ways in which intermediate processes occur has been sufficiently explored so that the routes through which household factors affect nutritional status may now be incorporated into the discussion. These are the social practices and biomedical linkages that are located in-between as it were. They exist and have their effects within household and community contexts; hence, they are not invariate from situation to situation, but modified by context.

Thirdly, with a more nearly complete picture before us, some reflections may be offered concerning how certain strategic parts of the whole system that produces health could be viewed. These reflections will be selective, chosen because they touch on issues that this research has highlighted.

Relating Household Resources to Nutritional Status

Following a procedure very similar to that used earlier, clusters of household resources may be represented by a parsimonious set of independent variables and the health outcome by a dependent variable, in this instance nutritional status.

Household income can be used this time, because its dating is similar to that of the health status of the child; both are current. So income is used to represent material resources. For schooling experience of the mother, a dichotomy for her years of education is used. Some other alternatives were considered to incorporate the husband's contributions, but they added little to the model of relationships.

An additional variable is brought into the investigation this time: the sanitation conditions of the household. It is dichotomized between whether the home has a complete system (tap in the dwelling or building plus a sewer connection) or not. With the additional understanding we now have of the relationships between sanitation and various intermediate factors, this variable will be of interest. Finally, a variable representing the social composition of the household is included. It is the same as before with three categories: complex compositions, simple compositions, and the female single-parent families that have households of their own.

Children's requirements for healthy growth, resistance to disease, and illness care are highly age dependent. Consequently, one expects the relationships between resources at the disposal of households and the health status achieved for children to have somewhat different structures as age increases. This raises the question of where to draw an arbitrary age boundary for the statistical modeling. Though the changes in requirements by age are continuous, there is a considerable difference between infancy and the second and third years of life which suggests an age boundary at that point in time. So long as it corresponds approximately with the actual requirements of children, using this boundary will bring out differences in how requirements are met as children grow older.

From earlier investigation, it is already known that nutritional status falls rather rapidly during the first year of life and is relatively stable across the

Table 7-1. Household resources affecting nutritional status: linear regressions for infancy and for second and third years of life

	During infancy		Second and third years	
Variables	Mean[a]	Coeffi-cient	Mean[a]	Coeffi-cient
Dependent				
Nutritional status (ratio of child's weight to median standard)	.971		.899	
Independent				
Continuous variable				
Household income in LE per month	160.0	.2-E3	165.2	.2-E3**
Categorical 0/1 variables [b]				
Mother's schooling experience (less than 5 years)				
5 years or more	.200	.023	.189	.028*
Sanitation system (incomplete or no sanitation system)				
Both tap and sewer	.164	.058*	.180	.002
Household composition (complex)				
Simple household	.825	.006	.852	.037*
Female single-parent family living alone	.036	.104	.056	.036
Statistics				
Constant	.922		.835	
R square	.036		.034	
Adjusted R square	.018		.022	
Number of children	275		412	

Significance: *p<.05; **p<.01. One-tail T-tests.

a. For categorical 0/1 variables the mean is the proportion giving a positive response.

b. For categorical variables, the coefficient is the difference in nutritional status associated with this category compared to the reference category shown in parentheses.

second and third years. It is also known that there are no detectable sex differentials. Variables for both age and sex were included in some of the models that were constructed, which confirmed the earlier findings.[1] For the sake of parsimony they are not included now, and the focus is on the other variables for which there are expected relationships to health status. The regression models, one for infancy and one for the second and third years, are shown in Table 7-1.

The first suggestion seen in the two regressions is that the influence on child growth of the household's material and social resources changes when children pass from infancy to the second and third years of life. The two statistical descriptions are quite different from each other. The influence of all the household resources is positive for both infancy and the second and third years of life, but statistical significance varies. Sanitary conditions of the home have a statistically significant and substantial influence (coefficient) on nutritional status during infancy but not afterwards. The other resources are not statistically significant during infancy, but acquire significance following infancy when their measured effects (coefficients) are also substantial.

The process that appears to account for the change reflected in the two statistical descriptions is one already known from earlier investigation, but one which can now be placed in the context of household resources and explored further.

At the beginning of life, children are protected against infection by passive immunity received from mothers and by anti-infective factors in breastmilk, but these decline, and as children begin to move around the house as well as receive food from external sources to meet their growth requirements, the exposure increases. We have also noted that even those children who are said to be breastfeeding exclusively receive small amounts of liquids and 'tastes' of other food from very early. Thus, the risk of transmission of infections to these children is more serious if the sanitation system of the household is incomplete and home hygiene poor. Until children become toddlers and move out into the community, their own household's situation is paramount. This suggests why household sanitation systems, if present, have a substantial beneficial effect on growth during infancy, whereas subsequently they do not appear to confer a relative advantage.

The heightened importance of household income, maternal education, and household composition as the child grows older is likely related to changes in the growth requirements of the child and the ability of household resources to support its needs. To understand how these social processes come to be so important, we need to reconsider the routes by which various resources of the household affect nutritional status.

Intermediate Routes by which Action and Process Affect Health Outcomes

Clues to the changing relevance of particular household resources during the first three years of life may be found by linking resources to child feeding patterns, prevalence of illnesses, and treatment practices. The nature of these linkages also suggests why they have less influence on child health in the setting of the Manshia during infancy and more influence later on.

By the second year of life, the most vulnerable children have died. Additional children will fail to survive the second and third years, but most will be 'survivors'. Resistance to some types of disease has been acquired and continued survival without deterioration is the question for them.

When examining linkages between social contexts and actions, we are not interested simply in demonstrating the likelihood that there is a predisposition to take certain actions when a particular resource is present. We are also interested in the growth consequences of the actions, and will try to show that actions have variable implications for the growth of children across households depending upon the different resource configurations that are present. In other words, implications of actions are context specific and thus the health consequences of particular behaviors are variable depending upon the social context in which they occur. For example, hygienic practices are indeed facilitated where there is better sanitation and more income. In addition, when children in this environment are taken off the breast after infancy, they do better than those still breastfeeding. Thus, resources and specific conditions of household life interweave with intermediate factors at the next level and affect the outcome.

One may draw the general conclusion that specific actions are often variable in their strength, because their effects depend upon the general context, which is itself defined by the resources of the household. This conclusion supports the now widely accepted idea that pediatric recommendations about home childcare should be tailored to the contexts in which they are going to be implemented. In order to do such tailoring, one needs the kind of information that we have tried to extract from this study of children of the Manshia.

Effects of the sanitation system on disease and hygienic practices

When one looks for reasons why parasite loads are so high and diarrheal illness is so frequent, the systems that people use for securing water and disposing of human waste must be implicated. The relationship of a household's sanitation system to prevalence of disease has been examined from a number of angles. One of the findings was that families were able to employ better hygienic practices when they had both tap water and sewerage than when one of these was absent. Attack rates of diarrhea were also lower by 22 percent in such households.

The connection between sanitation and health was also seen when infants who are receiving supplemental food or who have gone off the breast entirely were studied. These are a group of children believed to be at greater risk of disease, and therefore at risk of growth retardation. The comparison shows that children in homes with adequate sanitation were 13 percent more likely to have better nutritional status than infants in other homes, looking only at children receiving outside (non-breastmilk) foods.[2]

The full health benefits of water and sewer connections are not achievable by the individual household on its own. As children begin to move around, a high proportion of households in the locality need to be equipped with sanitation infrastructure and to be implementing good hygienic practices before an individual mother's diligence can be effective in bringing down the prevalence of parasitic disease and diarrheal illness.[3]

Income

Although household income does not show a statistically significant relationship to nutritional status during infancy (it does for the second and third years), probing by some additional procedures shows how it becomes an influential element of the household context. As mothers begin to use external sources of food besides breastmilk to feed their infants in mid to late infancy, income clearly becomes relevant to growth.

The income effect was identified by separating the infants into two groups, those in households with above median and below median income, and comparing within each type of household those infants who were only breastfeeding with those on supplemented or fully non-breastmilk diets. The infants who were only breastfeeding were found to have similar nutritional status regardless of their income class. However for those who were supplementing or not breastfeeding at all, nutritional status was significantly better for those infants living in richer homes.[4] The difference between rich and poor shows itself also in another way; there is no statistically significant deterioration in weights among infants living in higher income households when breastmilk is terminated during infancy, but there is in poorer households.

The meaning of these findings is that breastfeeding during infancy, as we have found it in the setting of Manshiet Nasser, insulates infants and makes them 'equal' in the face of economic differences. However, as they go off the 'natural' biological support provided by readily available mother's milk and need wider support from such specific factors as better environmental and personal hygiene, and need good food supplements, the economic resources of households make a difference. Thus, the critical period of weaning through which each infant must pass appears to be a less life-threatening period for those in richer homes.

In the second and third years of life, the regression shows a stronger and significant relationship of income to nutritional status. Another way of examining the route by which income influences nutritional status is to ask whether excessive durations of breastfeeding are related to poor income. The duration of breastfeeding—that is, when it is finally terminated—shows no significant relationship to income. Thus, continuation to very long durations, when it occurs, is probably not a practice related to women being very poor and substituting their own breastmilk for other food. Such extremes of poverty appear to be rare or non-existent in any event.

One way that income has implications for growth in the second and third years of life is through its effect on the diet of the family as a whole. Very few children are reported by mothers to be only breastfeeding after infancy whether in poorer or richer households. Since children are fed non-breastmilk foods mainly from the *tabliya* (family table), the quality of family food is a significant factor for their health. To the extent that a minority of children pass through a period when they receive specially prepared foods, their nutrient qualities may also be influenced by income.

The way that income mediates the effects of weaning on health, and contributes to better growth beyond infancy, should not be seen solely, or even mainly, as by the purchase and feeding of better food. Income is also associated with better hygienic physical environments which reduce exposure to infection. Income is also the basis for purchasing a variety of other assets that enhance the household environment: stove, refrigerator, soap, and more abundant supplementary water.

Schooling experience of mothers

Attention has been drawn repeatedly to the fact that schooling is a relatively rare experience among mothers in this settlement area. In spite of the limited schooling experience, the young children of educated mothers sustained better weights than those of uneducated mothers, particularly when children survived beyond infancy. While educated mothers do tend to live in households with higher incomes and better sanitary facilities, which are themselves environmental factors of the household that favor better health, the data described by the regression show that there is a distinct contribution by the mother's schooling experience; it is seen in infancy, without statistical significance however, and shows more conclusively as the child ages.[5]

One means by which educated mothers ensure better health for their children appears to be through more effective control of infectious diseases. The incidence of diarrheal illness is much lower among young children of educated mothers. The children of educated mothers had 25 percent less diarrhea than the children of uneducated mothers controlling for the level of incomes and the presence of sanitary facilities. Underlying the lower incidence of diarrheal illness is better control of hygienic aspects of home life. Soap was found in 25 percent of homes with educated mothers but only in 9 percent of homes with uneducated mothers. The difference by educational experience remained when income was controlled such that whereas educated mothers were four times as likely to have soap in the home when household income was above the median, they still were twice as likely to have it when poor.

The benefits that educated mothers can give to their children pass through the route of diet as well. While almost all mothers breastfeed their children, educated mothers tend to complete weaning earlier: seventeen months for less and fifteen months for more educated mothers (estimated at the mean). Since these durations far exceed the minimum necessary for healthy growth, the earlier completion by educated mothers could be contributing to more satisfactory growth.

More educated mothers also start the transition sooner than those with less schooling, giving solid foods to their children at earlier ages. We estimate that the mean age at which solid foods are started is 9.4 months for the less educated mothers and 8.1 months for the more educated.[6] Whereas there are less educated mothers still waiting to introduce solids as late as seventeen months, there is not a single educated mother who has not given solids by the age of nine months. The educated mothers clearly do better at modifying diet to keep pace with the changing requirements of children, a transition that is critical for growth at this stage in their young lives.

Household compositions

It was argued earlier, when we first looked at the social composition of households in Chapter 3, that the management of family resources on behalf of children by mothers is likely to be more effective when the residential arrangements accord the mother more undivided responsibility and autonomy in carrying out her maternal functions. We are now able to say that this is supported statistically in several ways. First, it was shown in Chapter 4 that mortality rates are better in households where the household is composed of both parents together with their children and no one else. Now we may add that a similar observation emerges when quality of survival, as measured by nutritional status, rather than survival itself is examined. Children in simple nuclear households have better nutritional status than in other households, after adjusting for other variables. With respect to single parenting, the children seem to do better also, but not as much so as those in simple nuclear-family households where both father and mother are present.[7]

One of the ways in which household compositions, and what they imply about the mother's managerial role, has an effect on nutritional status is through diet. The data suggest that once breastfeeding is terminated, the children living in simple households tend to maintain better nutritional status than those living in complex households, controlling for the effect of other resources.

A further route is by differences in therapy for children who have fallen ill. The children in simple households are taken more often for professional consultation when ill with diarrhea than children of other households.

This discussion of the health implications of different household compositions should not be interpreted as an argument for unqualified superiority of simple household living arrangements. Efficacy in the performance of the mothering role may be realizable in other household settings as well. There are aspects of the complex household that are beneficial to child health such as the possibility of higher income due to multiple earners, and the opportunity to mobilize more help, advice, and emotional support for home and childcare. The question is to what extent and in which ways, the negative and positive aspects of different household compositions are balanced with respect to child health in a given social and cultural setting. If we approach household environments in their multiple dimensions as dynamic systems producing health, rather than attempting to identify universally best levels or categories for each household resource, then we do find interesting clues in the information from the Manshia.

The health implications of specific household compositions vary depending upon the availability of the other household resources. That is to say, child health improves in both types of households when there is an improvement in sanitary conditions, in the mother's education, and/or (to a lesser extent) in the level of household income, but by different amounts.[8] When any of the household resources is improved, the gain in nutritional status is strongest in the complex households. However, when the general situation is one of poor resources, the simple households are able to maintain better nutritional status for their children (standardized weights average 91 percent of the norm in simple compared with 85 percent in complex households at equally poor levels of resources).

Complex households have larger numbers of members and are thus likely to have greater difficulty maintaining hygienic environments. It is notable, therefore, that having the resource of a complete sanitation system makes more difference for children's health than the same advantage in simple households. Education is another resource with differential effects. Women in simple households have more autonomy over daily management of their homes and children due to residential nucleation, irrespective of education. However, when women in complex households are able to gain such autonomy through the strength of their personal resources, which include education, they seem to be able to turn the greater resources of the complex household to advantage. This is seen by their having healthier children than educated mothers in simple households.

EIGHT

Reflections on Urban Growth and Health

While the study has focused mostly on one community, Manshiet Nasser, it has drawn attention to Cairo's larger fabric as well. One gains some understanding of the larger city by situating Manshiet Nasser in its Cairo setting. Life in Cairo at any particular time is shaped by the concerns and actions of families living in their own varied neighborhoods who are at different stages of household formation and integration into the city. It is the intersection of these household and community histories that recreates Cairo daily. The study of Manshiet Nasser provides us with one view into the dynamic of urban growth in this complex city and its meaning in terms of the health and welfare of its residents.

Forces that Create New Neighborhoods in Cairo

It is virtually certain that the demographic forces that are causing expansion in the settled areas of Cairo will continue in the future. Economic forces are more volatile, but they too appear to be following a similar trajectory. Thus, many additional neighborhoods will be built and settled. They will occupy unbuilt space shown on the map of Chapter 1, and push boundaries out further into the desert as well as on agricultural land. Existing built areas will become more and more densely settled.

During the 1980s, the pace of family reproduction was such that the number of dwellings was doubling every twenty-five years. One could detect in the demographic trends of fertility and mortality the seeds of a decline in that pace, but only slowly. Our projections, which are necessarily less certain the farther they reach into the future, suggest that the momentum will last, with a declining speed, until the mid-twenty-first century. The only questions that seem to be open are precisely where, at what pace in each specific instance, and with what standard of housing and community life new areas of the city will be settled. So there will be more Manshiet Nassers.

How fast this happens is largely set by the trends of fertility and early childhood mortality, with a time lag of twenty to twenty-five years. Fortunately for the gains in human welfare that it implies, mortality rates have been dropping rapidly. This was seen in the data for Manshiet Nasser as well.[1] Fertility is also declining, and its rate of decline has overtaken the decline of mortality. Families want fewer children because they know that most of them will now survive. Families have also been incorporated into the changing culture of Cairo that values education, with all the attention that needs from parents, and into forms of work and consumerism that require additional investments by the family in each new member. Thus, the logic of family formation decisions in Cairo is taking fertility down steadily, and this logic extends to families in the new neighborhoods.

Even though there will be continuing demographic pressure for new residential space, it will let up gradually. The largest benefit of the declining fertility and mortality is realized immediately in terms of less wasteful reproduction by families, particularly women who bear the pregnancies, births, and rearing responsibilities. The other major benefit is time lagged; the building of new settlements can eventually happen more slowly, giving more scope for families to acquire and organize resources for the conduct of daily life in these new areas.

Economic conditions also play a role. One channel through which they have an influence on Cairo's growth is migration. As the Egyptian economy is restructured by its own industrialization toward urban sites for production, which includes the myriad branches of service industries, the shift in locus of labor markets encourages migration to the cities. However, Egypt now has many cities with economic potential in Upper and Lower Egypt, so Cairo need not be a primary destination for such migration. Economic policies can influence the locational distribution of urban growth, marginally at least. Economic conditions in the international labor markets to which Egyptians have access are also influential as destinations for long periods of the working life of men.

For about a decade, from the boom in employment opportunities occasioned by the end of war in 1973 and the spectacular rise of demand for manpower in the Gulf states and Libya that followed, people were able to mobilize more material resources for business and families. Our survey caught Manshiet Nasser at the end of this boom period, just as the crest of better income opportunities for people of the lower middle and working classes was passing. A decline followed, and as we write in the early 1990s, a serious recession, possibly indicating a long term structural insufficiency of employment, exists in all of Egypt and in Cairo.[2]

Despite the decline in economic means, however, the demographic momentum of inter-generational reproduction will not go away. When squeezed, people respond by postponing plans for marriage while they are still young, but not indefinitely; eventually they act by making sacrifices in other areas of consumption in order to marry and to house themselves. They accept less ambitious housing objectives. To what extent the current stringency, and what may follow in the future, will affect the ability of households not only to reproduce, but also to rear healthy children, raises a serious question. Certainly, more income is better and less is likely to have adverse effects on health. This has been shown.

What Self-help Can and Cannot Do

It should be recalled that the city's formal systems, public and private, were no match for the rate of expansion in habitations demanded as long ago as the founding of the Republic in 1952. The crisis became an important agenda item for the socialist government of Nasser. An attempt was made to ensure that housing would be affordable for the middle and lower classes by instituting rent control and organizing public housing projects. There were many problems inherent in both parts of this two-pronged approach by the state, even though it clearly benefitted some classes of the population, though not others, for a time.

Inherent problems might have been endured, but the sheer scale of the housing that was being demanded soon overwhelmed the state system. By the 1970s the insufficiency began to be recognized, even at high levels of government, and economists were busy setting out the reasons why the formal system had either to be modified or abandoned and replaced by something new (Wheaton, 1980). Meanwhile the people themselves were fully aware of the failure as it touched them and were busy devising ways of coping at an individual family level.

For young adults needing homes, and their parents in alliance with them, the chosen route was, in most instances, to use informal processes outside the plans and controls of government to construct and to rent housing. While rent control and the building standards of city planners remained in force, ingenious ways were found at the informal level that would reward private builders adequately to make construction worthwhile, and renters would trade on the side with 'key money' to transfer dwelling units in an otherwise frozen market for existing housing. As these practices quietly became commonplace, they tended to replace formal systems, ushering in an era of predominantly informal building and the creation of whole self-help communities.[3] The systems that people used to do this were not entirely new; they already existed among small groups of migrant or poor families, but were a precarious, low-visibility form. With the increase of scale, the self-help system became dominant and highly visible. It has become a sustainable modern urban form, not some traditional rural transplant.

Through oral histories, a survey in 1984, and subsequent observation and in-depth studies in Manshiet Nasser, we have before us a history of thirty years for one of the new neighborhoods, and can ask how well the system works. Many of the needs of this community have been met eventually at some level, but some critical ones are still waiting. An ordering of when specific needs were met would show that those which could be addressed directly by residents through their own individual efforts, particularly housing, kept pace with the increase of residents in the settlement. Furthermore, the community did not have to wait long for small-enterprise private services such as retailing, doctor's clinics, and water delivery. Money demand brought prompt supply responses.

In addition to absorbing people as residents, Manshiet Nasser received the spill-over of growth in nearby workshop industries. It was close at hand, had inexpensive space, and was informal. This concurrent absorption of commerce and industry made an important contribution to the community by providing employment and cash inflow. All of this happened informally without benefit of formal institutions.

The settlement also provided for its own governance by setting up an informal system to resolve conflicts, maintain order, and to negotiate on its behalf with formal authorities. For more than thirty years of the Manshia's history, the Arab Council and the *'umda* provided a system of locally arranged governance on many matters, though it has now been outrun by the growth of the community and the demise of its charismatic leader. Eventually, the city absorbs the community into its own system of governance.

Slower to come into place were services that could not be organized by individuals or small groups. When the required scale of capital or household participation was large, or regulatory measures were needed, it was necessary to wait. Self-help did not readily extend itself to voluntary organizations with formal charters either. Such organizations have long been regulated by strict government controls and perceived as restrictive rather than supportive. Recently some signs of reorientation of public policy have been seen, but the historical experience has shaped many people's expectations. An exception is welfare activities based on formal religious institutions; they function under different regulations. For example, mosque and church-related programs have undertaken socially valuable community work including health services.

Since the experience of people has been that they usually can accomplish more by remaining informal, they have nurtured informality through their own social networks. Indeed, the networks are preferred over formal market and administrative systems in so many ways that the latter tend to fulfill skeptical expectations by remaining less developed. Consequently, some problems genuinely in need of municipal organizations, or large private organizations to reach solutions have been lacking. Such organizations exist, particularly in the older parts of the city, but their pace of extension to the Manshia has taken much longer than the self-help processes.

An exception was solid waste collection. A system was organized on behalf of the entire community at the beginning of the 1980s. A private formal organization was created, owned by a group of workers from the garbage collection industry. It serves the householders of the Manshia who are themselves more or less compelled to use it by collective social pressure. Another exception was electricity, where the public organization was flexible about the informal status of the community and prompt about extensions. In other areas of service needs, things moved more slowly.

What has just been said is not limited to physical infrastructure. It applies also to some elements of the social infrastructure. Schooling is an example. Expansion in educational facilities there has been (see above in Chapter 2), but always far behind requirements. The children of the Manshia are not entirely trapped, however, by this limitation. Many families go outside the Manshia and into Cairo to obtain schooling for their children.

One should understand that all urban services, social and physical, face tremendous demands for expansion everywhere in the cities of Egypt. Although population growth is slowing, the momentum will bring at least a further doubling to Egypt, and absorption is focussed on the cities. Thus, new settlements such as Manshiet Nasser have to fight for their place in the system of priorities of city and national government.

Under these circumstances, it is not too surprising that many officials have for long seen the informal settlements as nuisances to be pushed aside or eliminated; others have been willing to accept them but had little background or experience concerning how to do so. Few have seen them as places where clever solutions are found that might be supported. The predominant mood of officials has been to ask for total compliance with zoning and building codes as a precondition for provision of public services. There was a conflation of traditional urban planning precepts and the need to do something to ration demand for services.

Urban area upgrading came to Egypt in the 1970s on a wave of international attention to informal settlements. Perhaps the most significant contribution of the projects for area upgrading and sites and services that followed was not their specific accomplishments, which were limited, but the discussions that surrounded project negotiation and follow through, such as it was. These projects helped to set in motion more general recognition of these settlements as the present and future communities of the city. In the 1980s there were also projects for massive capital infusions into citywide infrastructure; they also had to face in one way or another the question of what to do about the new settlement areas. Thus, the standing departments of government and related public service organizations have been pressed to recognize the reality of these communities.

Meanwhile, the people of the self-help communities argue for accommodation. They have learned that solutions can be found by interlacing the formal and informal. As if to show that the informal process does not cease once formal services are in place, local residents make repairs to electric lines, fix sewage and water breaks, and assess each other in small groups for the expenses.

Patience and deprivation are a price that the self-help communities pay, believing firmly that at some point they will obtain the result they seek. Their own growth in scale and their people's desire to participate in more conveniences put new needs on the list, so negotiation with the formal authorities continues. In this regard, the new communities gradually become like older neighborhoods, all incorporated into the administrative politics of Cairo.

Child Health in New Neighborhoods

We started this study by taking the position that the health of children is both a component and an indicator of human welfare at the family and community levels. We have shown that many factors contribute to the human welfare outcome. Among them are the community's assets in terms of physical infrastructure, social infrastructure, and proximity to employment opportunities. At the family level, the assets of each household include such things as its dwelling, education and experience of the members, its system of internal organization, and income. All of these are inputs to the production of a welfare level. The inputs are not themselves direct measures of the welfare result, because the inputs must be used and transformed within the household and community first of all. It is this transformation, or production process, that produces healthy persons, in particular bringing health to the children who have been the focus of this study.

It is usually accepted that the achievement of health is aided by medical technologies and medical services available in the present day. However, to understand why many families, and particularly their children, can live in cities as rich in the availability of technology and services as Cairo, yet show ill health in many respects, one must look to the social context.

It was common in most cultures in past times to view illness as an imbalance in the relation between the individual and the environment, conceived broadly to include, physical, social, and supernatural elements. The development of modern medicine during the nineteenth century had the effect of separating the individual from the milieu by introducing a view of illness which located its causes in the malfunctioning of some part of the physiology of the individual. Accordingly, the task of medicine was redefined as acquisition and accumulation of a body of specialized knowledge with the aim of enabling its practitioners to locate the malfunctioning part and to fix it. This approach to illness both facilitated and gained strength from technological advances in methods of identification and treatment of diseases. It also placed concern with health exclusively in the domain of the medical profession.

These developments led to displacement of interest in health viewed as a process inextricably embedded in everyday life with an interest in illness conceived as episodic breakdowns of a physical mechanism. Under the dominance of this view, the consideration of the ways in which health is produced and reproduced within structures of daily life received much less attention. There have increasingly been reactions to abstraction of health issues from their social and cultural context.[4] The present study was conceptualized as part of such a reaction. We have argued throughout the analysis that the resources available to communities and to households, and the actions by which these resources are transformed in the course of sustaining daily life are the critical issues in understanding and thus improving the health and welfare of people. This is particularly the case for people whose health is threatened cumulatively from birth onwards by insecurities of employment, relative poverty of incomes, and inadequacies of physical and social infrastructure.

The study has sought to contribute to the formulation of a new understanding of health issues built on the insights of modern medicine but enriched by social analysis of the ways in which health is being produced as part of community and household life in today's specific settings. According to this perspective, health should not be seen as the exclusive domain or responsibility of health professionals or institutions. It is also the consequence and test of how well other social institutions are functioning. Identification of the non-medical aspects of life that have major health consequences, and endeavoring to understand how they affect the health of individuals, has been a central goal of this study.

With such a perspective, we came to the subject of the new neighborhoods looking for the conditions underlying family welfare and, in particular, child health. Young, newly-formed families of the vast lower and lower middle classes are settling these areas and creating the material and social environments where most of the next generation of Cairenes is being reared. The engine of growth of the Cairo population is overwhelmingly located in these neighborhoods. They are neighborhoods where multiplicity of rural backgrounds intermingle with the older culture of Cairo creating new urban forms, socially and physically.

What kind of human environment is being shaped in these communities? How are families coping with the insecurities of employment, constraints of low incomes, absence of a variety of public services? What are the implications of life in these neighborhoods for the health and welfare of the people living in them, particularly the children? These are the questions which led us into pursuing diverse lines of inquiry and into using multiple methodologies while exploring one particular fast growing area on the edge of Cairo. To understand the conditions and the quality of survival in this community, we sought for clues in the history of its formation as well as in the current lives of its residents. The result is one account, mainly through the health of its children, of the struggle for life in this dense and resilient city.

Notes

Chapter One

1 For an account of the bifurcated morphology of Cairo, native and foreign, see Abu-Lughod (1965; 1971). Her deservedly famous book is an excellent source for the development of the city of Cairo from its beginnings in the tenth century up to the mid-1960s.

2 For measurements and a discussion of the changes taking place, see Ibrahim (1987) and Shorter (1989).

3 The crude birth rate (births divided by total population) rose temporarily during the mid to late 1970s. Divergence from the downward trend of the total fertility rate was due to an unusual increase in numbers of women entering their twenties (and marriage), which is the time in their lives that childbearing rates are highest. This was one of those age-distribution effects. It was exaggerated by a slowing of the rate of decline in total fertility as well. With demobilization after the 1973 war, men re-entered the marriage market, many of them with money in hand as labor markets were buoyed by better wages at home and jobs in the Gulf.

4 The claims have probably been exaggerated, but there is no doubt that awareness among families of the possibilities for giving better care has been enhanced by stimuli and examples from many quarters. Deaths from all causes have declined, not only deaths that could be attributed to diarrhea alone.

5 For an essay that takes a long historical view and comments with insight on changing lifestyles in contemporary Cairo, see Nawal el-Messiri Nadim (1989).

6 Induced abortion is not accepted as legal in Egypt except for a narrow range of reasons, so its prevalence tends to be hidden from statistical view. Its existence as a secondary procedure when contraception fails and to assist women who have had clandestine abortions with medical complications is documented in hospital records, but these are a poor guide to prevalence.

7 The temporary reversal of trend that is seen for 1975–80 is traceable to those same causes that are mentioned in note 3 above. When the rate of decline in the total fertility rate slowed, it was temporarily overtaken by a rapid decline in mortality rates (see the infant mortality rate in Table 1-2).

8 Living arrangements following marriage and while bringing up a family are discussed in the chapter below on households (Chapter 3).

9 To make this comparison, past experience needs to be compared with a series of appropriately-dated net reproduction rates in the last column of Table 1-3. Since the table is not carried back to the earlier years, an element of rough estimation

is necessary to make this statement. Higher mortality in that earlier period probably held the NRR close to a constant level not much higher than 2.0, despite higher fertility.

10 The definition is by Castells and Portes (1989) in their introductory chapter to a valuable book on the analysis of the informal economy worldwide.

11 For a discussion of some of the differences among settlements, see Oldham, el-Hadidi, and Tamaa (1987).

12 For a discussion of the issues of comparability, scaling, and things left out, see Kelley (1991), as well as the candid self-assessment by the authors in the latest UNDP report itself (UNDP, 1991). See also Mukherjee (1989).

13 For studies of the age-pattern of mortality, and its systematic co-variation at all ages, see the literature on construction of model life tables. An authoritative work is Coale and Demeny (1983) and its earlier editions.

14 The age patterns of mortality are also similar in a general way across cultures, but there are differences. These are reflected in the demographic profession's use of what are called 'regional' models of mortality, each somewhat different from the others, that are graduated within each region by level (severity or force of mortality).

15 For a further explanation of the relationships and use of terminology, see Martorell and Ho (1984) and Mata (1978).

16 For a discussion of evidence from a broad range of disciplines that there is a two-way synergistic relationship between physical health and psychological well-being of children, see Myers (1992: Chapter 9).

17 The literature in Egypt on child development is scanty, though better can be expected in the future. The regional research program of the Population Council (MEAwards) is supporting efforts to develop concepts and operationalize their measurement for medium and large-scale surveys. Three investigators in particular may be mentioned: an anthropologist who is studying how mothers perceive and act upon child development in Egypt, Hania Sholkamy; and two social psychologists with extensive survey experience who have created and tested survey instruments in Turkish that can measure children's development from soon after birth to age six years, as well as some of the more important home environment variables that are influential, Işık Savaşır and Çiğdem Kağıtçıbaşı.

18 When MacLeod returned several years later, she found that the employee bus service had been extended to Dar es-Salam, which indicates how settlements are gradually recognized and brought into the urban system. Karima was commuting to work mornings by bus and leaving her children during the entire week, overnight included, with her mother in Sayyida Zeinab. She goes to them each afternoon and returns home in the evening by train as before (MacLeod, 1991:24–27).

Chapter Two

1 See map previous chapter; location code is (1).

2 He is not an *'umda* in the legal sense, since the term refers to village headmen who are appointed by the central government, an office that never existed in urban places. The powers of an *'umda* have been circumscribed considerably since the 1952 revolution. They used to be chosen from among the most influential people in the village community and performed a variety of administrative tasks

including resolution of local disputes. In terms of his leadership position and function in this urban community the leader of Manshiet Nasser was considered to be an *'umda* in the old village style.

3 There have been cases of persons who took quite substantial portions of land, a thousand square meters or more, both at the outset and subsequently. Some of these lands are only now being subdivided and sold at high prices. The general pattern of land development, however, was quite different from that seen in some other rapidly growing self-help areas. In these other places, middlemen staked claims to substantial tracts of publicly owned land, and then subdivided and sold off plots for construction. This type of large-scale land speculation was not seen in Manshiet Nasser, although profits on the increase of land values have certainly been made.

4 It is difficult to untangle the land tenure situation from oral accounts due to community insecurity regarding its legal status. Even today there is some insecurity about tenure, so that people are anxious to present what they think is the best picture of the way in which they acquired their land although they are unsure of what that might be. Some who did actually pay insist that they took their land without paying for it, in the belief that the law against trading in government land applies to the buyer as well as the seller. Some argue the opposite with the hope of reducing charges for tenure in case there is regularization of status.

5 The title transfer document for buildings states: 'I, [name], hereby sell my house built on land owned by the government to [name].'

6 In the case of one plot purchased in about 1980, for instance, sixty square meters of land were purchased for LE 700. Subsequent expenditures to level the ground reached LE 2,000, and thus the final investment was LE 45 per square meter. To some extent these costs are balanced by having to invest little in building foundations since the rock is solid enough to support high buildings with little concrete and steel as compared to that needed on agricultural land.

7 John Turner (1967) characterizes as 'progressive development,' the process whereby 'families build their housing and their community in stages as their resources permit, the more important elements first.' Houses and communities are lived in while they are built and modified as resources accumulate and the needs of the family cycle change. He contrasts this with the 'instant development' model which officially requires that minimum standard structures and community installations be in place prior to occupancy. Furthermore, little modification is allowed; people should move to another community when their needs change.

8 The owner's standard of habitability was accepted. If the official housing standards were applied most of these units would be classified as under construction (not finished) rather than as vacant.

9 A favorable attitude toward upgrading of existing settlements came into vogue among international assistance agencies and some governments in the 1970s, following a long period when demolition was seen as the answer to undesirable housing. For the rationale of this policy change, see Gilbert (1986) and an influential contribution to the attendant controversy by Turner (1967, 1968).

10 For a rich exposition of how networks of family, neighbors, and mid-level political processes function in Cairo on behalf of important needs that families have, see Diane Singerman (1989).

11 EQI undertook the project to demonstrate an affordable and sustainable approach to Cairo's garbage problems (EQI, 1982). It did so on behalf of the Governorate of Cairo. The experience gained has strengthened the institutions and organizational capacity of the Zabbaleen garbage collectors themselves. They now have a variety of systems for gathering garbage which they use as inputs for their recycling businesses.

12 The plastic containers are shaped like the steel containers for petrol that were known as 'Jerry cans' during the Second World War. In Cairo, the plastic ones are called *jerkins*.

13 Average storage of 270 liters would need 5.4 *jerkins* (fifty liters) six times per month for an average cost of LE 0.25 x 5.4 x 6 = LE 8.10 per month.

14 Hoda Sakr's Ph.D. dissertation (1990) provides the best documentation of the World Bank project and insight into how it was managed.

15 A contraceptive prevalence rate is the number of women currently practicing a method of contraception, including male methods, divided by the number of women who are married and between the ages of fifteen and fifty.

16 The 1991 estimates are preliminary findings of the Egyptian Survey for Mother and Child Health (PAPCHILD) conducted in early 1991 by CAPMAS in cooperation with the Arab League. The 1984 figures are from the Egyptian Contraceptive Prevalence Survey of that year.

17 The data have been moved from 1984 to mid-year 1985 by a projection procedure. Thus, the labels of 1985 still refer to the survey population, but with an adjusted date that compares well with other data.

18 The projection is made from the age and sex composition of the survey population with assumptions as follows. The trends of fertility and mortality in metropolitan Cairo are extrapolated to 2010 at rates similar to those in the past (Shorter, 1989). Then the levels of fertility and mortality for Manshiet Nasser (Table 2-6) are moved parallel to those of Cairo, keeping a differential between Cairo and the settlement. There is no migration in the projection. We are assuming that TFR will reach 3.5 children and the expectation of life at birth will reach sixty-eight years in Manshiet Nasser by 2010. This could be unduly conservative (pessimistic); however, changing the assumptions to a more rapid transition has very little effect on the size of the young adult population up to the year 2010.

19 From a tabulation of the 1988 Egyptian Demographic and Health Survey which was conducted by the Egyptian National Population Council.

20 This computation is based on six schools with the capacities that were planned when the building projects were started, namely fourteen rooms in each school with a capacity of forty-five students per room. Subsequent adaptation may have made it possible to enroll more students, but we could not confirm this.

21 See, for example, *Egyptian Gazette*, February 6, 1989.

22 This quantity is derived from the increase in women of childbearing ages by natural increase alone, excluding the increase due to migration, shown in Figure 2-3, and the quantity will increase more rapidly after the year 2000.

23 We are indebted to Heba el Kholy for an unpublished paper that illuminates this question, 'Towards a typology of women-headed households in low income communities: suggestions from field research in Egypt,' presented to the Population Council's Working Group on Family Resources, June 1990.

24 Dr. Saneya Saleh kindly provided information about the Society and other aspects of education and social services in Manshiet Nasser.

25 For an early application of Polanyi's typology of exchange systems (reciprocity, redistribution, and market exchange) to an urban setting, see Lomnitz's (1974) study of life in a squatter settlement in Mexico City. A recent study of how the urban poor use social networks to manipulate the system in relation to daily needs and housing in a large city on the Turkish Mediterranean coast is by Duben (1991). For other neighborhoods of Cairo, see the articulate and detailed study of the heart of old Cairo by Singerman (1989: Chapter 3), as well as the valuable studies of Nadim (1977) and Hoodfar (1988: Chapter 9).

Chapter Three

1 Many of the ideas and concepts in this section were developed during an earlier collaboration with Huda Zurayk on the social composition of households in Arab cities and settlements (1988, 1990). We particularly want to acknowledge the fruitfulness of that association.

2 We are indebted to Dr. Ahmed for discussions that elaborated on her empirical findings. Her study is based on a representative sample of households interviewed as a follow-up to the 1980 Egyptian Fertility Survey.

3 We are indebted to Dr. Gürsoy-Tezcan for allowing us to cite this information from her unpublished work, part of which is available as Gürsoy-Tezcan (1992).

4 A study from Latin America shows that the nutritional status of children is affected adversely when the mother lives in a consensual union rather than a formal marriage, the interpretation being that the husband's commitment is weaker and resource pooling less effective. However, the same type of analysis was performed comparatively for West Africa and yielded no adverse effect on nutritional status for children of polygamous as compared with monogamous marriages (Desai, 1991). Indeed, the resource pooling and other aspects of family functioning are complex and no doubt culturally specific.

5 The literature on families with only one parent offers a variety of terminological possibilities. By single-parent, we mean one parent is present, without implying anything about marital status. We avoid the term 'broken' most of the time, even though used just now to suggest a prior transition.

6 A similar figure, but different in details, was first suggested by Ermish and Overton (1985) in an entirely different context—the demand for housing in Britain. They partitioned households into "minimal housing units" according to the conventions of British society concerning who might live with whom. Then they noted how these minimal units of persons might move off to separate housing, or recombine in households of more than one minimal unit—useful for studying housing demand.

7 A good source for the European experience, with extensive references is Wall, Robin and Laslett (1983). For contemporary Britain see Ermish and Overton (1985). Many of the same questions arise and are dealt with in an important study of the Muslim population of Istanbul at the turn of the century (Duben and Behar, 1991).

8 That was true in 1984, but the government began soon after to let the queue of eligibles become longer and longer without actually hiring the applicants. Then, in the late 1980s it canceled this 'right' of graduates.

9 For literature in the English language, see for example the novels of Naguib Mahfouz or stories of individual women by Nayra Atiya (1984). A serious scholarly study that bears out the drama is Singerman (1989).

10 In the sample of 1118 households, there were no unmarried females living alone. Elsewhere in Cairo, it is practically the same; the citywide sample found only three unmarried women living alone.

11 Refers to married women aged 25–49. The lower age boundary minimizes the bias, if any, that might be due to under-representation of late marrying women. (Source: Tabulations of the 1980 Egyptian Fertility Survey). The same age boundary is observed for the Manshiet Nasser estimate that follows.

12 In her study of an old, but also 'poor' area of Cairo, Andrea Rugh (1984), says that the wife's point of view favors marriage to her mother's sister's son, because it strengthens mutual support among females. But from the husband's point of view, the woman should marry her father's brother's son, strengthening male control and management of the extended family system. The male view is the one usually cited as the prevailing cultural preference in Egypt, not surprisingly.

13 The experience of and preference for different types of marriage systems has generally been discussed in terms of their implications for economic and political advantage and in particular for inheritance of property. For discussions of their relevance to the nature and meaning of intra-group relations, particularly between spouses and among females who have multiple links, see Fischer (1978), Dwyer (1978), Wikan (1982), and Abu Lughod (1987).

14 Mothers-in-law are found in 23 percent of the complex households, and the mother of the wife herself in another 7 percent. (One complex household in the sample gave a home to both the husband's and the wife's mothers!)

15 Husbands average eight years older than wives. Widowhood rates are directly increased by the age difference due to the higher life-table probabilities of dying of husbands compared with wives. This is additional to the more moderate difference in expectation of life for men (lower) than women at any particular age.

16 In the previous chapter, in relation to social infrastructure, the activities of private voluntary agencies that concern themselves with such households were mentioned.

17 Work in the Arab countries is the main reason. It is customary for men to be away on contracts of at least a year; usually they chain their contracts or jobs and stay longer. Many of them visit home once a year taking advantage of religious holidays that are recognized for purposes of leave in the Arab countries.

18 An ethnographic study in low income areas of Giza, and a mini-survey, carried out by H. Hoodfar and Fatma Khafagy in 1986, documents the points of view of women and shows how they manage during the long absences of husbands (unpublished drafts kindly made available). Also see Fergany's national survey findings (1988, 1989).

19 Mothers also tend to have more children with them, an average of 2.5 compared with 2.0 children for fathers.

20 Sahar el-Tawila has developed a methodology for tackling this problem, but it requires retrospective life-history information concerning women's successive states of marriages and dissolutions, along with information about the children living with them at each stage. An application based on incomplete information

from a national household and fertility survey in Egypt is made in her Ph.D. dissertation (1990), also reported in el-Tawila and Sayed (1991). It shows that the probabilities of ever being divorced, separated, or widowed, and of being a single-parent are certainly higher than our estimates show, but her estimates can only suggest broad ranges. Until surveys with the necessary questions are conducted in Egypt, we have to be content with drawing attention to the problem but not knowing its true scale.

21 For a reliable and sensitive discussion of the relationships of women and men with regard to work and cash earnings, see Nadim (1977).

22 Indeed, by the 1980s, civil servants were being called the 'new poor' of urban Egypt (Hansen and Radwan, 1982:127). In public-sector enterprises, the situation was less serious but worse off than the private sector.

23 The poverty line is defined as a level of income sufficient to meet minimum dietary requirements and minimum needs for housing and basic goods.

24 Korayem has two 'poverty lines', one at LE 150 and the other at LE 183, which we have used. The difference reflects assumptions about food prices. The second includes a cost factor for the use of intermediaries to gain access to rationed and subsidized foods, which was common in Manshiet Nasser in 1984, the date of her estimates and ours. Since then, government shops have become more accessible to people in the settlement, which lowers the poverty line and raises more people in the Manshia above it.

25 Private lessons have become widespread in Egypt at all levels of the educational system and among all classes of society, both urban and rural, constituting what some observers call a parallel system of education. The parents are willing to pay substantial sums, which increase as one goes up the educational ladder, to obtain individual or small-group instruction to help their children pass end-of-year examinations, particularly at those junctures when the examination alone is the gateway to the next higher level of the system. Many parents believe that tutorials by the classroom teacher are necessary to ensure satisfactory grades. On the supply side of tutoring are the teachers whose salaries have not kept up with the rate of inflation or with rising levels of living in Egypt, so they are only too willing to earn additional income in amounts that usually far exceed their salaries. Due to rapid expansion in the demand for education, and the limitations of the public educational system quantitatively, qualitatively, and financially, parents and teachers, together with some freelance tutors, maintain this informal education sector (Singerman, 1989:208–11; Waterbury, 1983:234–41).

26 The average size of each type of household, counting everyone equally, is shown above in Table 3-1.

Chapter Four

1 Methods developed by W. Brass (Brass and Coale, 1968) and elaborated since then (United Nations, 1983:73-85) are used to convert the crude measures into precisely defined life-table indices such as the proportion of children born who die up to age two, three, or five. For an introduction to the methodology, the UN reference is generally accessible. For the present study, mortality rates were estimated separately for the children of mothers grouped into three marriage durations, 0–4, 5–9, and 10–14 years. In order to increase the robustness of the

final estimates, the results for the three groups were combined. A 'West' model life table was selected on this basis to represent infant and early childhood mortality in this community. Indices for the population dying up to various ages of early childhood are used in the present study; they are all derived from a single representative model life table selected as just explained. See Table 4-1 above.

2 See comprehensive article by Gordon *et al.* (1963), which effectively questions the usefulness of concentrating on infant mortality worldwide as 'the accepted measure of general accomplishment in public health.' The article makes the point that while in industrialized countries infant mortality is a valuable index, in less developed countries it alone is not sufficient. This is because the death rates do not decline as sharply immediately after infancy but only after the second year of life so that infant mortality 'fails adequately to reflect that important part of health difficulties which comes into play at a later date, and depends heavily on the malnutrition associated with weaning after breastfeeding and during the immediately subsequent months' (p. 377).

3 UNICEF (United Nations Children's Fund) and some of the other international agencies that report health indices have recently begun to use the proportion dying up to age five (${}_5q_0$) as a measure of 'child mortality'. While the choice of age five rather than the true turning point in survival rates, which is closer to completed age three, is less than optimum, it is nevertheless superior to using infant mortality uncritically.

4 To make this comparison we have to express the Cairo rates in terms of the same index, i.e. the proportion dying up to age three. The basic statistical data for Cairo are from the vital registration system with which one estimates infant mortality rates directly. We extrapolate those rates to proportions dying under age three by using an appropriately selected model life table to represent the age-pattern of mortality in this particular instance.

5 Details of the differentials may be found in Shorter (1989:14–16). The basic study on this question was by Batani (1982) and referred to Cairo governorate.

6 The most common would be a move of the mother with her child (or children) from a complex household to a simple household of her own after having one or more children. Such moves within the Manshia are not numerous; most of them are from households in Cairo to the Manshia. (Children's living arrangements were discussed in Chapter 3). The statistical assignment of the current living arrangement to the woman would have the effect of attributing her children's survival experience to simple households rather than complex ones. As will be seen below by comparing survival in the two settings, the measurement bias would be to reduce, not enlarge, the differential for complex and simple households, provided transitions from one household to another are not selective with respect to child mortality which they probably are.

7 Another type of transition poses no problem. Eight women among the 414 in the sample are currently living with their husbands without any children. In seven of these cases, a child had been born but died (in one instance two born and two died). The deaths apparently precipitated the transition from a simple household with children to a simple household without children for each of these women. Since the woman is assigned as living in a simple household, which is a category that includes both the type before and after transition, no error of attribution is

generated. The eighth woman had been married eight years; her child is still alive and living elsewhere. It is not known whether the early years of life of this child's life were spent in a simple household or not, although that is the higher of the two probabilities and the survival experience is so classified.

8 In her study of the determinants of what she terms 'death clustering' Monica Das Gupta (1990) adjusts statistically for one factor after another, giving particular attention to women's autonomy, social class, and mothers' education. Ultimately she squeezes out an unexplained element of 'clustering' and attributes that to 'the basic abilities and personality characteristics of the mother (or other primary caretaker)' (p. 505). This conclusion might be unfair to the mothers involved, but it does point to the possible value of going further in field work and making measurements of what social psychologists term competence and efficacy.

9 A primus stove is a single-burner device that uses kerosene under pressure by a hand pump.

10 Unlike standard regression models, MCA imposes no assumption about the form of the relationship (whether linear or non-linear) of the dependent variable, the mortality rate, to each of the independent, socioenvironmental variables. It is particularly suited, therefore, to analyzing the effect of categorical variables such as those used in the study. It also tolerates association among independent variables.

11 The effects shown in the table have plus and minus signs that relate the numbers to the grand mean. To calculate spread, one effect is subtracted from the other.

12 The term 'single-parent' does not necessarily indicate a civil status of unmarried, but only that one of the parents is not currently residing in the household for whatever reason.

13 There was also a technical reason for constructing the combined variable. To maintain the assumptions of an additive model, interaction could be eliminated by making this combination.

14 Combining in one variable is also technically necessary to avoid an unacceptable level of interaction in the MCA.

Chapter Five

1 For a discussion of criteria for choosing among anthropometric indices for specific problems in analysis of nutritional status, see Bairagi (1985). His study identifies weight-for-age as the best indicator for assessing factors that affect nutritional status with medium and long term effects. Therefore, weight is an appropriate choice when both of the variables—weight and age—can be measured well under field conditions. We believe that this was accomplished in the Manshiet Nasser survey.

2 Several international standards exist. For the historical record we would like to note that the Harvard standards give virtually the same statistical results as the NCHS standards, in all but one respect. They expect somewhat higher weights for girls in the second, and especially the third, years of life than the NCHS standards. As a result the Harvard standards appear to detect a small amount of 'sex discrimination' against girls in the Manshiet Nasser sample when, according to the NCHS standards, none exists.

3 The reference curves are smooth, showing normal cumulative growth, except for a small 'hesitation' at age twenty-four months. It is not normal for growth to stop

or reverse for a month at the end of the second year. The hesitation appears to be due to a change in composition of the reference population at the beginning of the third year of the study that was used to establish the NCHS standards (our hypothesis). The 'wiggle' was retained by the scientists concerned, rather than smoothed over, underlining the point that no standard is perfect.

4 The NCHS standard is constructed so that medians and means are the same.

5 Those children who die disappear from the data and do not appear at older ages in the chart. This is a selection factor which tends to limit the downward trend of the curve. It also contributes to the upward drift of the curve during the second and third years of life.

6 The first survey was carried out between January and April 1978 and the follow-up survey was carried out during months when diarrheal diseases are more prevalent, August and September, in 1980. The prevalence of undernutrition measured by weight-for-age was higher in the 1980 survey, which is attributable to the season, but the age pattern of undernutrition remained the same.

7 This estimate is based on the EDHS estimate for Alexandria and Cairo governorates combined of 7.8 percent and for all urban places of 8.9 percent. It is necessary to interpolate because no separate estimate was reported for metropolitan Cairo.

8 If one looks at the trend within the first six months, growth retardation has started. See Figure 5-3.

9 The evidence from field-based studies concerning the effect of nutritional status on resistance to infection is mixed. While there is good evidence that poor nutritional status is associated with more severe episodes of infection, particularly the diarrheal, it is not clear that malnutrition predisposes to more frequent attacks. Some studies have found infectious diseases to occur more frequently among malnourished children (Scrimshaw *et al.*, 1968; Tomkins, 1981; el-Samani, 1985) while other studies found no association (Chen *et al.*, 1981; Black *et al.*, 1984). There is also the problem that where an association is found it may be confounded by socioeconomic factors; infection and poor nutritional status may tend to occur together because they are both consequences of poor living conditions, but are not as much causes of each other as appears statistically.

10 Diarrheal illness was identified by asking whether the child experienced three or more loose or watery stools in a day during the past two weeks.

11 The prevalence of diarrheal illness (in percent) on the day of the survey by age groups (in months) of children is as follows: (0–5)=14; (6–11)=21; (12–17)=18; (18–23)=12; (24–29)=13; (30–34)=7; and (all ages)=15.

12 Although information on seasonality of diarrheal disease is difficult to find in Egypt, it is commonly accepted that January through April is the period of low incidence, whereas July through September with its hot summer weather is the high period. The diarrheal prevalence found in two national nutrition surveys carried out at different seasons of the year (one in January–April 1978 and the other in August 1980) seem to confirm the generally accepted pattern. A study of diarrheal deaths over a one year period in Menufiya governorate indicated a primary peak during June through September, which is consistent, and a secondary peak in November-December, which has not otherwise been remarked upon in the Egyptian literature (Tekçe, 1982).

13 It has been observed that the incidence of lower respiratory tract infections, primarily pneumonia and bronchiolitis, decreases with age (Foster, 1984). We do not know what proportion of the acute respiratory illnesses reported by the mothers were of this type. It is known however that lower respiratory tract infections tend to account for a much higher proportion of the acute respiratory infections in the Third World countries as compared with the developed countries (*Lancet*, 1985:699–701).

14 Infection refers to entry of an infectious agent followed by its development or replication in a host. Superinfection occurs when a host acquires more parasites of the same type before the initial infection dies. This is a particularly important process for helminthic infections (worms), because they do not reproduce in quantity within the body except by being re-ingested. Their health consequences are dependent upon the intensity (quantity of worms) of infection. In the case of asexual replicating organisms such as protozoa, multiplication occurs within the host. Therefore a heavy infection can develop within a few days or weeks after the initial infection which may be a single agent or many organisms depending upon what constitutes an infective dose for a given pathogen. For a discussion of these issues, see Mosley (1980), Feachem *et al.* (1983), and Bradley and Keymer (1984).

15 This age pattern was found in a study of urban living conditions of five squatter communities in Amman, Jordan (UDD, 1982). The same timing of infestation was also documented in detail in Mata's Guatemala study (1978).

16 The sample was taken in May. Parasite prevalence rates are much less affected by seasonality than other illnesses, because they are acquired over time and continue thereafter to live in the human host unless treated.

17 The fecal specimens were preserved and stained with the M.I.F. solution and the preserved specimens were examined microscopically using the concentration technique.

18 Assessment of items in adult diets is a very difficult task and was considered beyond the scope of this study. Therefore the detailed composition of diets for children who were reported to be partaking wholly or regularly from family diets was not investigated.

19 A report on one of the participant-observation activities of this research was published by Oldham (1984).

20 In a detailed study of the determinants of infant mortality in Malaysia, the authors found that the lower mortality of breastfed children during infancy was primarily a function of the duration of exclusive breastfeeding. Their findings indicated that the infants who were fully breastfed during the first month had lower mortality both during that month and in the next five months regardless of the feeding mode in the subsequent months. See DaVanzo *et al.* (1983) and Butz *et al.* (1984).

21 For an extensive description of the tasting process in rural Upper Egypt where many of the Manshia's mothers come from, see the studies by el-Hadidi (1990) and Sholkamy (1990).

22 The estimate of timing is made by using the information on whether the child is currently receiving solid foods by age of the child. The mean age at which solid foods are given is estimated by the current status method to be 9.2 months.

23 In an excellent discussion of child feeding practices and nutrition in tropical and subtropical countries, Jelliffe notes the uncertainty concerning the actual optimal

length of breastfeeding and observes that: 'As an approximate gauge it is advised that breastfeeding be continued up to at least one, and preferably two years, according to local circumstances.' (Jelliffe 1968:168). Morley is even more definite and states that: 'The two years of breastfeeding . . . is probably the normal period for *homo sapiens* as a mammal.' (Morley 1978:101).

Chapter Six

1 For well-documented materials on the central role of mothers in Cairo's lower income communities see Atiya (1984), Rugh (1984), Hoodfar (1986), Nadim (1989), and Oldham (1991).

2 For assistance in identifying transmission routes and other epidemiological characteristics of parasitic disease, we particularly want to acknowledge Professor W. Henry Mosley's interest and support.

3 A study of living conditions in self-help settlements located inside the city of Amman, Jordan, found that the Giardia rates were higher for families with access to water main connections when compared to those without and suggested that the cysts may be distributed through the municipal water system (UDD, 1982:101).

4 A comprehensive report on environmental hazards to health was prepared based on examinations of living conditions and stool samples of 12,000 persons living in thirty-five villages of Egypt (Miller, 1981). It emphasizes repeatedly that the single most important transmission route for intestinal parasites and diarrheal agents may be the household water containers (*zir*). Although water storage is a necessity in Manshiet Nasser, the practice of storing drinking water has a long history in Egypt. Drinking water is customarily stored in unbaked porous pots which cool the water by slowly 'sweating' their content. These are found in homes irrespective of the availability of piped water and also in the streets for public use. A study of the bio-chemical quality of water stored in the *zir* in a village in the delta where all households had both piped water and latrines, found that 34 percent of the samples contained parasitic and bacterial contamination (el-Sebaie *et al.*, 1981).

5 *E. histolytica* infection seems to be endemic in Egypt. A survey among students aged fifteen to twenty years found the prevalence of cyst excretion to be 16 percent in the Nile Delta and 11 percent among those in Upper Egypt (Arafa *et al.*, 1978, cited in Feachem *et al.*, 1983:339).

6 For an interesting discussion of how the immediate neighborhood functions as if it were an extension of family space rather than public space, see Nadim (1977).

7 Also reported in Oldham (1984:30–32).

8 In a study in urban Bangladesh it was found that simply providing soap to families with instructions on hand washing could reduce the transmission of bacillary dysentery by more than 75 percent among persons within a household who were in contact with an infected person (Khan, 1982). For a detailed review of studies on hand washing and transmission of pathogens see Feachem (1984).

9 The statistical model was the same as that shown in Table 6-1 except that the dependent variable is whether or not a diarrheal illness was experienced during two weeks prior to the survey.

10 As in the previous multivariate models, independent variables for mother's education and household income are included to filter out their effects via intermediate variables on nutritional status. It is recognized that a layered

statistical model would be technically superior to examine the hypothesis, but an adequate number of observed variables for this purpose are not at hand. This multiple linear regression gave a p-value of 0.004 for the sanitation variable. Details of the modeling are in Tekçe (1990:935).

11 The relevant statistical analysis is given in the next chapter for two- and three-year old children.

12 For a series of studies that have been particularly illuminating in this regard, we would note the surveys and reports made by Sarah Loza of SPAAC, a consulting firm, to the National Control of Diarrheal Disease Project (NCDDP). See also Sholkamy (1992).

13 Medical education in Egypt is in English, and doctors frequently speak in English in front of patients. More importantly, there is cultural distance, which the patients recognize. For example, among other types of diarrheal syndromes there is one which the mothers in the Manshia call *nazla sha'biya*. This diarrheal illness may or may not be accompanied by vomiting and fever but involves colored stools. To the parents it means a diarrheal illness which is caused by living in a popular (low-income) quarter: *sha'b* means people. Doctors also use the term but in a completely different way to mean bronchitis, derived from the word *shu'ab*. Doctors consulted on this point acknowledged that poor people frequently mispronounce the term, but they were not aware that a different meaning is intended.

14 Treatment of diarrheal illness shows a statistically significant age pattern with infants receiving more care than older children (chi-square = .004). This difference arose mainly from differences among male children (chi-square = .01). Infant females also received more professional attention than older female children but the difference was not statistically significant (chi-square = .14). Professional consultation for respiratory illness, on the other hand, does not show statistically significant differences by age or sex.

15 The differential treatment of ill children by sex is more pronounced in the case of diarrheas. The information on severity enabled us to disaggregate the care behavior to show that the sex bias occurs strongly in the case of simple diarrheal episodes. There is a slight tendency to seek advice from professional sources more for boys in respiratory illness as well but because no confirmation was collected on severity it is not possible to examine the relationship of this bias to severity of illness. In terms of seeking advice from sources outside the settlement, the sex differential is again more pronounced in the case of diarrheal than respiratory illness. Proportions using doctors outside the settlement or hospitals during diarrheal illness were for boys .49 and girls .27; and during respiratory illness were for boys .38 and girls .36.

16 Makinson's sample of 1613 children aged under five years who were admitted to a Cairo oral rehydration center during August 1983 to July 1984 showed that more males than females were admitted for treatment, but that girls were more likely to die at the rehydration center than boys. She also reports the anomalous finding that no difference in symptoms or health status by sex was recorded upon admission, which she suggests could be attributed to poor measurement.

17 Controlling for education of the mother shows that in households where the mother has less than five years of schooling (most of them), the division is practically the same: 57 to 39 percent (Chi-square significant at .029).

Chapter Seven

1 There is a suggestion in cross-tabulations of the data that the positive effects on nutritional status of more income, more mother's schooling, and simple household compositions are greater for girls than boys. Thus, if there is any discrimination against girls, it disappears when household resources are favorable. In an analysis of variance, for example, the direction of net effects marginally favors girls, not boys, but the magnitude is trivial and not statistically significant. The detection of sex differentials, when small, is also sensitive to the choice of the nutritional standard. See note 2 of Chapter 5.

2 The relationship was investigated by a regression model which included in addition to diet: sanitation, mother's education, and household income. It allowed for interaction of diet with sanitation. The diet variable was constructed by dividing infants into those who were solely breastfeeding and others who were receiving non-breastmilk foods partially or only. The difference that sanitation makes when infants are receiving outside foods (.128) has a *p* value of 0.003. The difference sanitation makes to the differential in standardized weights for the two categories of feeding (–.132) has a *p* value of 0.020.

3 This is the reason why statistical models that take households as units, all within a single community, do not show the importance of sanitation facilities after infancy even though it probably exists.

4 The procedure was to estimate the mean standardized weights by breastfeeding pattern from two regressions, one for children in households with above median income and one with below median income. Controls for other resource factors were included. The estimates were then compared by feeding pattern and tested for statistical significance. For poorer households, the effects are significant ($p<.02$), whereas there is no significant difference by feeding pattern in the richer households (Tekçe, 1990:935–36).

5 Though we are looking at nutritional status, it may be noted that the voluminous literature on relationships between parental education and child mortality generally reports a stronger effect of maternal education on death rates in childhood than in infancy, and this is confirmed by examination of the national data sets of the World Fertility Survey (Cleland, 1990). On the Egyptian WFS, see Makinson (1986).

6 As we have done elsewhere in this study, children of different ages are used to form synthetic cohorts to estimate the means. This avoids having to ask respondents to date past actions, which would introduce recall errors that are often serious.

7 The direction of the effect on nutritional status (Table 7-1) shows that the female single-parent formations are better than complex living arrangements, but the coefficient is not statistically significant, no doubt due to the small number of cases (N=23).

8 There are too few complex households to estimate meaningfully a model with all the extra interaction terms, including those for two separate periods of early childhood. Instead, we pooled all children under age three and reduced household composition to two categories: simple (including single-parent households) and complex. A separate regression for each category of household was used to evaluate the effect of the different resources on nutritional status. The results discussed in the text come from these two regression equations.

Chapter Eight

1 See in particular the downward trend of mortality implied by the slope coefficient of the variable for marriage duration in Table 4-2.

2 The onset of recession after the early *infitah* period and the gravity of the new employment situation faced in Egypt since then are set forth with excellent documentation and interpretation in a recent volume edited by Heba Handoussa and Gillian Potter (1991).

3 Among high-income people also, informal construction became commonplace, undermining formal procedures from the top as well as the bottom.

4 An excellent discussion of the recent developments in medical sociology in terms of both subject matter and perspectives is given by Bryan S. Turner (1987). He weaves together skillfully the analyses of Foucault, Navarro, Parsons, and interactionists and brings out the critical problems inherent in the medical model of illness.

Bibliography

Abt Associates, Dames and Moore, General Organization for Housing, Building Planning and Research. 1982. 'Informal Housing in Egypt.' Report to U.S. Agency for International Development.

Abu-Lughod, Janet. 1965. 'Tale of Two Cities: The Origins of Modern Cairo,' *Comparative Studies in Society and History*, vol 7 (1964–65), 429–60.

Abu-Lughod, Janet. 1971. *Cairo: 1001 Years of the City Victorious*. Princeton: Princeton University Press.

Abu-Lughod, Lila. 1987. *Veiled Sentiments: Honor and Poetry in a Bedouin Society*. Cairo: The American University in Cairo Press.

Aga Khan Award. 1985. *The Expanding Metropolis: Coping with the Urban Growth of Cairo*. Proceedings of a seminar held in Cairo, November 1984. The Aga Khan Award, Geneva.

Ahmed, Ferial Abd el-Kader. 1987. 'Fertility Transition in Egypt.' Ph.D. dissertation in demography, University of Pennsylvania.

Arafa, M.S., A.M.S. el-Ridi, H.D.A. Ezzat, and L.M. Makhlouf. 1978. 'A Seroparasitological Study of Entanoeba histolytica in Egypt', Journal of the Egyptian Society of Parasitology 8: 229–332.

Arriaga, E. and K. Davis. 1969. 'Patterns of Mortality Change in Latin America,' *Demography* 6: 223–42.

Assaad, Ragui. 1989. 'The Employment Crisis in Egypt: Trends and Issues.' Paper presented at The American University in Cairo, January.

Assaad, Ragui. 1990a. 'Structured Labor Markets: The Case of the Construction Sector in Egypt.' Ph.D. dissertation, Cornell University, Ithaca, New York.

Assaad, Ragui. 1990b. 'Informal Labor Markets: The Case of the Construction Sector in Egypt.' Paper presented at the 1990 annual conference of the Middle East Studies Association. New Orleans.

Assaad, Ragui. 1991. 'Structure of Egypt's Construction Labour Market and its Development since the Mid-1970s,' *Employment and Structural Adjustment: Egypt in the 1990s*, ed. Heba Handoussa and Gillian Potter. Cairo: The American University in Cairo Press. p 125–65.

Atiya, Nayra. 1984. *Khul-Khaal: Five Egyptian Women Tell Their Stories*. Cairo: The American University in Cairo Press.

Bairagi, R. 1985. 'A Comparison of Five Anthropometric Indices for Identifying Factors of Malnutrition.' Carolina Population Center, University of North Carolina at Chapel Hill.

Batani, Denise K. 1982. 'The Relationship Between Child Mortality and the Educational Status of Mothers in Egypt.' M.Sc. thesis, Department of Statistics, Faculty of Economics and Political Science, Cairo University.

Bibliography

Behm, H. 1979. 'Socio-economic Determinants of Mortality in Latin America.' Paper presented at the Meeting on Socio-economic Determinants and Consequences of Mortality, World Health Organization, Mexico City, June.

Berger, P. and T. Luckmann. 1967. *The Social Construction of Reality: A Treatise on the Sociology of Knowledge.* New York: Doubleday and Company, Inc.

Berman, P.A. 1982. 'Selective Primary Health Care: Is Efficient Sufficient,' *Social Science and Medicine* 16: 1054–59.

Birkbeck, C. 1979. 'Garbage, Industry, and the 'Vultures' of Cali, Columbia,' *Casual Work and Poverty in the Third World Cities*, ed. R. Bromley and C. Gerry. New York: Wiley.

Black, R.E., K.H. Brown, and S. Becker. 1984. 'Malnutrition is a Determining Factor in Diarrheal Duration, but not Incidence, among Young Children in a Longitudinal Study in Rural Bangladesh,' *American Journal of Clinical Nutrition* 39: 87–94.

Blum, D. and R.G. Feachem. 1983. 'Measuring the Impact of Water Supply and Sanitation Investments on Diarrheal Diseases: Problems of Methodology,' *International Journal of Epidemiology* 12: 357–65.

Bradley, D. and A. Keymer. 1984. 'Parasitic Diseases: Measurement and Mortality Impact,' *Child Survival Strategies for Research*, supplement to *Population and Development Review* volume 10: supp 163–87.

Brass, W. and A. Coale. 1968. 'Methods of Analysis and Estimation,' *The Demography of Tropical Africa*, ed. W. Brass. Princeton: Princeton University Press.

Briscoe, J. 1984. 'Water Supply and Health in Developing Countries: Selective Primary Health Care Revisited,' *American Journal of Public Health* 74, no. 9: 1009–1013.

Butz, W.P. , J.P. Habicht, and J. Davanzo. 1984. 'Environmental Factors in the Relationship Between Breastfeeding and Infant Mortality. The Role of Sanitation and Water in Malaysia,' *American Journal of Epidemiology* 119, no. 4: 516–25.

Caldwell, J.C. 1979. 'Education as a Factor in Mortality Decline: an Examination of Nigerian Data,' *Population Studies* vol 33: 395–413.

Caldwell, J. and P. McDonald. 1981. 'Influence of Maternal Education on Infant and Child Mortality,' in International Union for the Scientific Study of Population, *International Population Conference Manila*, vol 2. Liege.

CAPMAS. 1978. Central Agency for Public Mobilization and Statistics. *General Census for Population and Housing 1976: Detailed Results for the Whole Republic.* September, Cairo.

CAPMAS. 1987. Central Agency for Public Mobilization and Statistics. *First Preliminary Report on the 1986 Census.* April, Cairo.

Castells, Manuel and Alejandro Portes. 1989. 'World Underneath: The Origins, Dynamics, and Effects of the Informal Economy,' *The Informal Economy: Studies in Advanced and Less Developed Countries*, edited by A. Portes, M. Castells, and L.A. Benton. Baltimore and London: Johns Hopkins University Press. pp 11–37.

Centers for Disease Control. 1986. *CDC Standard Deviation-Derived Growth Reference Curves: Derived from the NCHS/CDC Reference Population.* Software V3.0 by Michael D. Jordan. Division of Nutrition, CDC, Atlanta.

Chen, L.C. 1986. 'Primary Health Care in Developing Countries: Overcoming Operational, Technical, and Social Barriers. *The Lancet.* Nov. 29: 1260–65.

Chen, L.C., E. Hug, and S.L. Huffman. 1981. 'A Prospective Study of the Risk of Diarrheal Diseases According to the Nutritional Status of Children,' *American Journal of Epidemiology* 114: 284–92.

Cleland, John. 1990. 'Maternal Education and Child Survival: Further Evidence and Explanations,' What We Know about Heal*th Transition: The Cultural, Social and Behavioral Determinants of Health*, ed. John Caldwell, Sally Findley, *et al.* 400–419.

Cleland, John and Jerome Van Ginneken. 1989. 'Maternal Schooling and Childhood Mortality,' *Journal of Biosocial Science* 10 (supplement): 13–34.

Coale, A.J. and P. Demeny. 1983. *Regional Model Life Tables and Stable Populations.* Second edition with Barbara Vaughan. New York: Academic Press.

Cochrane, S. 1980. *The Effects of Education on Health.* Washington, D.C.: World Bank, Staff Working Paper 405.

Cornia, G.A., R. Jolly, and F. Stewart. 1987. *Adjustment with a Human Face.* Vol 1. New York: Oxford University Press.

CPD Egypt Panel. Committee on Population and Demography. 1982. *The Estimation of Recent Trends in Fertility and Mortality in Egypt.* Report No. 9. US National Research Council. Washington: National Academy Press.

Crompton, D. and M.C. Nesheim. 1984. 'Malnutrition's Insidious Partner,' *World Health* (March): 18–21.

Das Gupta, Monica. 1990. 'Death Clustering, Mother's Education and the Determinants of Child Mortality in Rural Punjab, India,' *Population Studies* 44, no. 3 (November): 489–505.

DaVanzo, J., W.P. Butz, and J.P. Habicht. 1983. 'How Biological and Behavioral Influences on Mortality in Malaysia Vary During the First Year of Life,' *Population Studies* 37, no. 3 (November): 381–402.

Davis, K. 1956. 'The Amazing Decline of Mortality in Underdeveloped Areas,' *American Economic Review* 46: 305–318.

Desai, Sonalde. 1991. 'Children at Risk: The Role of Family Structure in Latin America and West Africa,' World Conference on Demographic and Health Surveys, August 5–7, Washington, D.C.

Doan, Rebecca Miles. 1988. 'Class and Family Structure: A Study of Child Nutritional Status in Four Urban Settlements in Amman, Jordan.' Ph.D. dissertation. Cornell University.

Doan, Rebecca Miles and Leila Bisharat. 1990. 'Female Autonomy and Child Nutritional Status: The Extended-Family Residential Unit in Amman, Jordan,' *Social Science and Medicine* vol 31(7): 783–89.

Duben, Alan. 1991. 'The Rationality of an Informal Economy: The Provision of Housing in Southern Turkey,' *Structural Change in Turkish Society*, ed. M. Kiray. Indiana University Turkish Studies No. 10.

Duben, Alan and Cem Behar. 1991. *Istanbul Households: Marriage, Family and Fertility, 1880–1940.* Cambridge Studies in Population, Economy and Society in Past Time. Cambridge: Cambridge University Press.

Dubois, R. 1979. *Mirage of Health: Utopias, Progress, and Biological Change.* New York: Harper and Row Publishers.

Dwyer, Daisy H. 1978. *Images and Self-Images: Male and Female in Morocco.* New York: Columbia University Press.

Environmental Quality International (EQI). 1982. 'Completion of the Manshiet Nasser Pilot Solid Waste Route Extension Program,' Final Report presented to the Governorate of Cairo, November.

Ermish, J.F. and E. Overton. 1985. 'Minimal Household Units: A New Approach to the Analysis of Household Formation,' *Population Studies* vol 39: 33–54.

Esrey, S.A., R.G. Feachem, and J.M. Hugues. 1985. 'Interventions for the Control of Diarrheal Diseases among Young Children: Improving Water Supplies and Excreta Disposal Facilities,' *Bulletin of the World Health Organization* 63, no. 4: 757–72.

Evans, J.L., G.A. Lamb, N. Murthy, and F. Shorter. 1987. 'Women and Children in Poverty: Reproductive Health and Child Survival,' Report to the Trustees of the Ford Foundation for its Mid-decade Review of Programs. New York: The Ford Foundation.

Feachem, R.G. 1984. 'Interventions for the Control of Diarrhoeal Diseases among Young Children: Promotion of Personal and Domestic Hygiene,' *Bulletin of the World Health Organization.* 62, no. 3: 467–76.

Feachem, R.G., D.J. Bradley, H. Garelick, and D. Duncan Mara. 1983. *Sanitation and Disease: Health Aspects of Excreta and Waste Water Management.* World Bank Studies in Water Supply and Sanitation 3. Chichester: John Wiley.

Fergany, Nader. 1987. *Differentials in Labour Migration, Egypt (1974–1984).* Occasional Paper No. 4, Cairo Demographic Centre.

Fergany, Nader. 1988. *Seeking Daily Bread: Field Study on Migration of Egyptians to Work in Arab Countries* (Arabic). Beirut: Center for Arab Unity Studies.

Fischer, Michael M.J. 1978. 'On Changing the Concept and Position of Persian Women,' in L. Beck and N. Keddie, *Women in the Muslim World.* Cambridge and London: Harvard University Press. pp 189–215.

Folbre, N. 1986. 'Cleaning House: New Perspectives on Households and Economic Development,' *Journal of Development Economics* 22: 5–40.

Foster, S.O. 1984. 'Immunizable and Respiratory Diseases and Child Mortality,' *Child Survival Strategies for Research*, supplement to *Population and Development Review* vol 10: supp 119–40.

Gerry, C. 1979. 'Small-Scale Manufacturing and Repairs in Dakar: A Survey of Market Relations within the Urban Economy,' *Casual Work and Poverty in the Third World Cities*, ed. R. Bromley and C. Gerry. New York: Wiley.

Gilbert, A. 1987. 'The Housing of the Urban Poor,' *Cities, Poverty, and Development*, ed.A. Gilbert and J. Gugler. Oxford: Oxford University Press. pp 81–115.

Gordon, J.E., I.O. Chitkara, and J.B. Wyon. 1963. 'Weanling Diarrhea,' *American Journal of the Medical Sciences* 245: 345–77.

Gürsoy-Tezcan, Akile. 1992. 'Infant Mortality: a Turkish Puzzle?' in Health Transition Review 2, no. 2: 131–149.

el-Hadidi, Haguer. 1990. 'Sociocultural Factors Influencing the Prevalence of Diarrrheal Disease in Rural Sohag,' Monograph series on Egypt, UNICEF. New York.

Handoussa, Heba and Gillian Potter (eds.). 1991. *Employment and Structural Adjustment: Egypt in the 1990s.* Cairo: The American University in Cairo Press.

Hansen, Bent and Samir Radwan. 1982. *Employment Opportunities and Equity in Egypt.* Geneva: International Labour Office.

Hasan, Nawal Mahmoud. 1986[?]. 'Social Aspects of Urban Housing in Cairo.' Presentation to the Aga Khan Award for Architecture Seminar on 'The Expanding Metropolis' held in Cairo, November 1984, pp 59–61.

Hobcraft, J., J.W. McDonald, and S. Rutstein. 1983. 'Child Spacing Effects on Infant and Early Child Mortality,' *Population Index* 49, no. 4 (winter): 585–618.

Hoodfar, Homa. 1986. 'Child Care and Child Survival in Low-Income Neighborhoods of Cairo,' *Regional Papers.* Cairo: The Population Council.

Hoodfar, Homa. 1988. 'Survival Strategies in Low-Income Neighbourhoods of Cairo, Egypt,' Ph.D. dissertation, University of Kent, United Kingdom.

Huffman, S.L. and B.B. Lamphere. 1984. 'Breastfeeding performance and child survival,' Child Survival: Strategies for Research, supplement to Population and Development Review, vol 10: supp 93–116.

Ibrahim, Mahmoud F.M. 1987. 'Features and Causes of Internal Migration in Cairo Economic Region,' M.A. thesis in demography, U.N.–A.R.E. Cairo Demographic Centre. Cairo.

Ikram, Khalid. 1980. *Egypt: Economic Management in a Period of Transition. A World Bank Country Economic Report.* Baltimore: The Johns Hopkins University Press.

Issawi, C. 1982. *An Economic History of the Middle East and North Africa.* New York: Columbia University Press.

Jelliffe, D.B. 1968. *Infant Nutrition in the Subtropics and Tropics.* Geneva: World Health Organization.

el-Kadi, Galila. 1987. *L'Urbanisation Spontanée au Caire.* Centre d'Etudes et de Recherches URBAMA à l'Université de Tours, Fascicule de Recherches No. 18, Tours.

el-Katsha, S., A. Younis, O. Sebaie, and A. Hussein. 1989. 'Women, Water, and Sanitation: Household Water Use in Two Egyptian Villages.' *Cairo Papers in Social Science*, vol 12: 2. Cairo: The American University in Cairo Press.

Kelley, Allen C. 1991. 'The Human Development Index: "Handle with Care",' *Population and Development Review* 17(2): 315–24.

Khan, M.U. 1982. 'Interruption of Shigellosis by Hand Washing,' *Transactions of the Royal Society of Tropical Medicine and Hygiene* 76, no. 2: 164–68.

Khouri-Dagher, Nadia. 1986. *Food and Energy in Cairo: Provisioning the Poor.* United Nations University Food–Energy Nexus Programme. Cairo: Institut Français de Recherche Scientifique pour le Développement en Coopération (ORSTOM).

Kielmann, A.A., and C. McCord. 1978. 'Weight-for-age as an Index of Risk of Death in Children,' *The Lancet.* 10 June: 1247–50.

Kielmann, A.A., I.S. Uberoi, R.K. Chandra, and V.L.Mehta. 1976. 'The Effect of Nutritional Status on Immune Capacity and Immune Responses in Preschool Children in a Rural Community in India,' *Bulletin of the World Health Organization* 54: 477–83.

Korayem, K. 1987. 'The Impact of Economic Adjustment Policies on the Vulnerable Families and Children in Egypt.' A report prepared for the Third World Forum, Middle East Office and the United Nations Children's Fund, Egypt. April.

Kunitz, S. 1987. 'Causes and Effects: Explanations and Ideologies of Mortality Patterns in Twentieth Century Epidemiology.' Paper presented at the Conference on Health Interventions and Mortality Change in Developing Countries, The University of Sheffield, Sheffield, 9–11 September.

Laslett, Peter (ed.) assisted by Richard Wall. 1972. *Household and Family in Past Time.* Cambridge: Cambridge University Press.

Lancet. 1985. 'Acute Respitatory Infections in Under-Fives: 15 Million Deaths a Year.' September 28: 699–701.

LeVine, Robert A., S.E. Levine, A. Richman, F.F.T. Uribe, C.S. Correa, and P.M. Miller. 1991. 'Women's Schooling and Child Care in the Demographic Transition: A Mexican Case Study.' *Population and Development Review* vol 17(3): 459–96.

Lloyd, Cynthia B. and Sonalde Desai. 1991. 'Children's Living Arrangements in Comparative Perspective,' World conference of Demographic and Health Surveys, August 5–7, Washington, D.C.

Lomnitz, L. 1974. 'The Social and Economic Organization of a Mexican Shantytown,' *Anthropological Perspectives on Latin American Urbanization*, ed. W. Cornelius and F. Trueblood. Latin American Urban Research, vol 4. Beverly Hills: Sage Publications. pp 135–55.

McKeown, T. 1976. *The Role of Medicine: Dream, Mirage or Nemesis.* Princeton, New Jersey: Princeton University Press.

McLanahan, Sara. 1985. 'Family Structure and the Reproduction of Poverty,' *American Journal of Sociology*, vol 90(4): 873–901.

MacLeod, Arlene Elowe. 1991. *Accommodating Protest: Working Women, the New Veiling, and Change in Cairo.* Columbia University Press, New York.

Makinson, C. 1986. 'Sex Differentials in Infant and Child Mortality in Egypt,' Ph.D. thesis, Princeton University.

Martorell, R. and T. Ho. 1984. 'Malnutrition, Morbidity, and Mortality,' *Child Survival Strategies for Research*, supplement to *Population and Development Review*, vol 10: supp 49–68.

Mata, L. 1978. *The Children of Santa Maria Cauque: A Prospective Field Study of Health and Growth.* Cambridge, Mass: MIT Press.

Meier, G. 1970. *Leading Issues in Economic Development: Studies in International Poverty.* New York: Oxford University Press.

Meier, G. and D. Seers. 1984. *Pioneers in Development.* London: Oxford University Press.

el-Messiri, Sawsan. 1978. 'Self-images of Traditional Urban Women in Cairo,' in Lois Beck and Nikki Keddie, *Women in the Muslim World.* Cambridge and London: Harvard University Press. pp 522–40.

Miller, F. 1981. 'Analysis of Environmental Data from Egyptian Rural Villages.' Report of research conducted jointly by the University of Michigan and Egyptian Academy of Scientific Research and Technology.

Moore, H.A., E. de la Cruz, and O. Vargas-Mendez. 1965. 'Diarrheal Disease Studies in Costa Rica: The Influence of Sanitation upon the Prevalence of Intestinal Infections and Diarrheal Disease,' *American Journal of Epidemiology* 82, no. 2: 162–84.

Morley, D. 1978. Paediatric Priorities in the Developing World. London: Butterworths.

Morsy, Soheir A. 1978. 'Sex Differences and Folk Illness in an Egyptian Village,' in Lois Beck and Nikki Keddie, *Women in the Muslim World.* Cambridge and London: Harvard University Press. p. 599–616.

Moser, C. 1978. 'Informal Sector or Petty Commodity Production: Dualism or Dependence in Urban Development,' *World Development* 6 (Sept.–Oct.): 1041–64.

Mosley, W.H. 1980. 'Biological Contamination of the Environment by Man,' *Biological and Social Aspects of Mortality and Length of Life*, ed. S.H. Preston. Liege: International Union for the Scientific Study of Population.

Mosley, W.H. 1983. 'Will Primary Health Care Reduce Infant and Child Mortality? A Critique of Some Current Strategies with Special Reference to Africa and Asia,' Seminar on Social Policy, Health Policy and Mortality Prospects, Paris 28 February–4 March. Paris: Institut National d'Etudes Démographiques (INED).

Mosley, W.H., and L. Chen. 1984. 'An Analytical Framework for the Study of Child Survival in Developing Countries,' *Child Survival: Strategies for Research*, supplement to *Population and Development Review*, vol 10: supp 25–45.

Mukherjee, Ramkrishna. 1989. The Quality of Life: Valuation in Social Research. New Delhi: Sage Publications.

Myers, Robert. 1991. *The Twelve Who Survive: Strengthening Programmes of Early Childhood Development in the Third World.* London and New York: Routledge in co-operation with UNESCO for The Consultative Group on Early Childhood Care and Development.

Nadim, Assad, Nawal Nadim, and Sohair Mehanna. 1980. 'Living Without Water.' *Cairo Papers in Social Science*, vol 3: 3. Cairo: The American University in Cairo Press.

Nadim, Nawal el-Messiri. 1977. 'Family Relationships in a Harah in Cairo,' *Arab Society in Transition: A Reader*, Saad Eddin Ibrahim and Nicholas S. Hopkins (eds). Cairo: The American University in Cairo Press, pp 107–120. Republished in *Arab Society: Social Science Perspectives*, Hopkins and Ibrahim (eds). Cairo: The American University in Cairo Press, 1985, pp 212–22.

Nadim, Nawal el-Messiri. 1989. 'Changing Lifestyles in Cairo,' *Urbanism in Islam*, Supplement, 112–28. The Middle Eastern Culture Center in Japan, University of Tokyo.

Nelson, J. 1969. 'Migrants, Urban Poverty, and Instability in Developing Countries,' Cambridge, Mass: Center for International Affairs, Harvard University, *Occasional Papers* 22.

NPC (National Population Council). 1989. *Egypt Demographic and Health Survey 1988.* Cairo.

Nutrition Institute, Ministry of Health, Arab Republic of Egypt. 1979. *National Nutrition Survey: 1978*, Cairo.

Nutrition Institute, Ministry of Health, Arab Republic of Egypt. 1980. *Nutrition Status Survey II: 1980*, Cairo.

Oldham, Linda. 1984. 'Child Nurturance and its Context at Manshiet Nasser, Cairo,' *Regional Papers*, Cairo: The Population Council.

Oldham, Linda. 1991. 'Case Management for Diarrheal Disease in Children under Age Three: An Ethnographic Study in Six Communities of Egypt,' Report by Social Planning, Analysis and Administration Consultants (SPAAC) to the National Control of Diarrheal Diseases Project (NCDDDP), unpublished, Cairo.

Oldham, Linda, Haguer el-Hadidi, and Hussein Tamaa. 1987. 'Informal Communities in Cairo: The Basis of a Typology,' *Cairo Papers in Social Science*, vol 10: 4. Cairo: The American University in Cairo Press.

Plank, S.J. and M.L. Milanesi. 1973. 'Infant Feeding and Infant Mortality in Rural Chile,' *Bulletin of the World Health Organization* 48: 203–210.

Portes, Alejandro. 1981. 'Unequal Exchange and the Urban Informal Sector,' *Labor, Class and the International System*, ed. A. Portes and J. Walton. New York: Academic Press.

Portes, Alejandro. 1984. 'Industrial Development and Labor Absorption: A Reinterpretation,' *Population and Development Review* 10, No. 2 (December): 589–611.

Puffer, R.R. and C.V. Serrano. 1973. *Patterns of Mortality in Childhood.* Washington, D.C.: Pan American Health Organization.

Rageh, A. 1985. 'The Changing Pattern of Housing in Cairo,' *The Expanding Metropolis: Coping with the Urban Growth of Cairo*, The Aga Khan Award for Architecture. Proceedings of Seminar Nine in the Series Architectural Transformations in the Islamic World, held in Cairo, Egypt, November 11–15, 1984.

Rugh, Andrea. 1984. *Family in Contemporary Egypt.* Syracuse, NY: Syracuse University Press.

Sabbour Associates. n.d. 'Manshiet Nasser Up-Grading: Final Report Part I Urban Planning,' Presented to Cairo Governorate. Cairo.

Sakr, Hoda. 1990. 'Underlying Collegial Relationships Controlling Project Implementation: Case Study of Egypt.' Ph.D. dissertation in Urban and Regional Planning, Massachusetts Institute of Technology.

el-Samani, Fatih. 1985. 'Associations of Malnutrition with Malaria and Diarrhea: A Community Study of Children in Rural Sudan.' Dissertation submitted to the Harvard School of Public Health.

Scrimshaw, N., C. Taylor, and J. Gordon. 1968. *Interactions of Nutrition and Infection.* World Health Organization Monograph Series no. 57. Geneva.

el-Sebaie, O., A. Khairy, L. el-Attar, and A. Gawad. 1981. 'The Quality of Drinking Water in ABBIS II Village: Chemical Assessment of 'Zir' Stored Water.' Paper submitted to the 17th Annual Meeting of American Water Resources Association, Atlanta, Georgia.

Sen, A. 1984. 'Ingredients of Famine Analysis: Availability and Entitlements,' *Resources, Values and Development.* Oxford: Basil Blackwell.

Sholkamy, Hania. 1990. 'Sociocultural Factors Influencing the Prevalence of Diarrheal Disease in Rural Assiut,' Monograph series on Egypt, UNICEF. New York.

Sholkamy, Hania M. 1992. 'What we Say and What they Know: Egyptian Peasants in the Context of Health Intervention,' *Towards More Efficacy in Women's Health and Child Survival Strategies: Combining Knowledge for Practical Solutions,* ed. Ismail Sirageldin and Robb Davis. Baltimore: The Johns Hopkins University School of Hygiene and Public Health. pp 113–29.

Shorter, Frederic. 1989. 'Cairo's Leap Forward: People, Households, and Dwelling Space,' *Cairo Papers in Social Science,* vol 12: 1. Cairo: The American University in Cairo Press.

Singerman, Diane. 1989. 'Avenues of Participation: Family, Politics and Networks in Urban Quarters of Cairo.' Ph.D. dissertation, Department of Politics, Princeton University; forthcoming Princeton University Press.

Stolnitz, G. 1955. 'A Century of International Mortality Trends: I and II,' *Population Studies* 1955 vol 9: 24–55 and 1956 vol 10: 17–42.

el-Tawila, Sahar. 1990. 'Models of Family Demography, a Case Study: Egypt.' Ph.D. dissertation, Faculty of Economics and Statistics, Cairo University.

el-Tawila, Sahar Ismail and Hussein Abdel Aziz Sayed. 1991. 'Patterns of Family Life Cycle and Household Structure in Egypt,' *Occasional Paper* no. VI, Cairo Demographic Center.

Tekçe, Belgin. 1982. 'Oral Rehydration Therapy: An Assessment of Mortality Effects in Rural Egypt,' *Studies in Family Planning* 11 (November): 315–27.

Tekçe, Belgin. 1990. 'Households, Resources, and Child Health in a Self-help Settlement in Cairo, Egypt,' *Social Science and Medicine* vol 30(8): 929–40.

Tekçe, Belgin and F.C. Shorter. 1984. 'Determinants of Child Mortality: A Study of Squatter Settlements in Jordan,' *Child Survival: Strategies for Research,* supplement to *Population and Development Review,* volume 10: supp 257–80.

Tomkins, A. 1981. 'Nutritional Status and Severity of Diarrhea among Pre-School Children in Rural Nigeria,' *The Lancet* (18 April): 860–862.

Trussell, J. and S. Preston. 1982. 'Estimating the Covariates of Childhood Mortality from Retrospective Reports of Mothers,' *Health Policy and Education,* vol 3: 1–36.

Turner, Bryan S. 1987. *Medical Power and Social Knowledge.* London: Sage Publications.

Turner, John F.C. 1967. 'Barriers and Channels for Housing Development in Modernizing Countries,' *Journal of the American Institute of Planners* 33: 167–81.

Turner, John F.C. 1968. 'Uncontrolled Urban Settlement: Problems and Policies,' *The City in Newly Developing Countries*, ed. G. Breese. Englewood Cliffs, NJ: Prentice Hall. pp 507–534.

United Nations. 1973. *The Determinants and Consequences of Population Trends: New Summary of Findings on Interaction of Demographic, Economic and Social Factors.* Department of Economic and Social Affairs, Population Studies No. 50. New York: U.N.

United Nations. 1983. *Indirect Techniques for Demographic Estimation: Manual X.* Department of International Economic and Social Affairs, Population Studies No. 81. New York: U.N.

United Nations Children's Fund (UNICEF). 1984. *The State of the Worlds's Children 1984.* New York: Oxford University Press.

Urban Development Department (UDD). 1982. 'A Baseline Health and Population Assessment for the Upgrading Areas of Amman.' A report to the UDD by the Population Council (L. Bisharat, W.H. Mosley, F.C. Shorter, B. Tekçe). Municipality of Amman, Hashemite Kingdom of Jordan.

United Nations Development Programme. 1991. *Human Development Report: 1991.* New York: Oxford University Press.

Wall, Richard (ed.) with Jean Robin and Peter Laslett. 1983. *Family Forms in Historic Europe.* Cambridge: Cambridge University Press.

Walsh, J. and K. Warren. 'Selective Primary Health Care: An Interim Strategy for Disease Control in Developing Countries,' *New England Journal of Medicine* 30, no. 18: 967–74.

Ware, H. 1984. 'Effects of Maternal Education, Women's Roles, and Child Care on Child Mortality,' *Child Survival: Strategies for Research* supplement to *Population and Development Review*, vol 10: supp 191–214.

Waterbury, John. 1983. The Egypt of Nasser and Sadat: The Political Economy of Two Regimes. Princeton, New Jersey: Princeton University Press.

Wheaton, William. 1980. 'Public Policy and the 'Shortage' of Housing in Egypt,' *Housing Working Papers 1979/80.* Cairo University–M.I.T. Technological Planning Program.

Wikan, Unni. 1982. *Behind the Veil in Arabia.* Baltimore: The Johns Hopkins University Press.

Winikoff, B. 1983. 'The Effects of Birth Spacing on Child and Maternal Health,' *Studies in Family Planning* 14, no. 10: 231–45.

Winikoff, B. and M.A. Castle. 1988. 'The Influence of Health Services on Infant Feedings,' *Feeding Infants in Four Societies: Causes and Consequences of Mothers' Choices*, ed. B. Winikoff, M.A. Castle, and V.H. Laukaran. New York: Greenwood Press.

Zurayk, Huda and Frederic Shorter. 1988. 'The Social Composition of Households in Arab Cities and Settlements: Cairo, Beirut, Amman,' *Regional Papers*, No. 31. Population Council, Cairo, 88pp. Shortened version in Arabic in *al-Mustaqbal al-'Arabi (The Arab Future)*, 12: 58–80, Beirut, 1990.

Index

Index